DAVIDSON
MEDICAL
SERIES

VOLUME I

PERITONEAL DIALYSIS

Editorial Contributors

Janet Bardsley, Joanne Bargman, Mary Brandt, Ingemar Davidson, Kendle Frazier, Maurizio Gallieni, Christine Hwang, Shawna McMichael, Anil Paramesh, Eric Peden, Ramesh Saxena, Daniel Scott, Douglas Slakey, Min Yoo

This publication is funded entirely by DIVADI LLC/Ingemar Davidson.

DAVIDSON MEDICAL SERIES

VOLUME I

PERITONEAL DIALYSIS

Surgical Technique and Medical Management

EDITORS

INGEMAR DAVIDSON

MAURIZIO GALLIENI

RAMESH SAXENA

DIVADI LLC, DALLAS, TEXAS

ISBN: 978-0-9845463-2-9

Correspondence:
Ingemar Davidson, MD, PhD
3824 Cedar Springs Road #199
Dallas, Texas 75219
drd@ingemardavidson.com

Web sites:
www.ingemardavidson.com
www.imslc.com
www.dialysiscontroversies.com
www.vascular-access.info
www.controversiesindialysis.org

CHAPTERS

FORWARD
by Dr. Robert N. McClelland

The new Davidson Medical Series details both technical aspects and enduring tenets in this emerging subspecialty of vascular access in end-stage renal disease and treatment of malignancy. The book and video series are an expansion on Dr. Davidson's book *Access for Dialysis: Surgical and Radiologic Procedures* and its second edition published in 2002.

Since the publication of the first edition in 1996, there have been several significant changes in the population of patients with end-stage renal disease and the products available for dialysis access. Patients entering treatment programs for end-stage renal disease are now significantly older, usually in the 6th decade, because people are living longer. In fact, it is not unusual to initiate dialysis in 90-year-old individuals. In addition, most patients often suffer from multiple co-morbidities, most notably diabetes, hypertension, obesity, and cardiac and peripheral vascular disease. The end-stage renal disease population poses a significant challenge to the vascular access surgeon, not just in the creation of an access, but also in the maintenance of its function and patency. In the two prevalent modalities, hemodialysis and peritoneal dialysis, technical advances in materials and design now provide the treatment team with more choices. The downside to these developments is an increasing number of products, often without stratifiable data on their usefulness. Also, interventional radiologists and nephrologists have joined surgeons in the vascular access arena with a wide arsenal of techniques and devices to maintain patency, survey for impending access failure, and correct access complications.

Within this framework of an increasing patient population, numerous products, additional practitioners and available treatment options, access for dialysis continues to attract attention from surgical institutions and training programs, individual surgeons, nephrologists, radiologists, patient advocacy groups and payers. As dialysis therapy continues to be refined, providing increased life span and quality of life, patients require more maintenance and repair procedures than creation of new access. The skillful management of access, over time, may have the greatest impact on long-term patient outcome on dialysis.

It is in this forum that Dr. Davidson's extensive surgical experience and thoughtful attention to detail are most prominent. The teaching of surgical procedures and techniques is presented in a clear, accessible format that can be utilized by experienced staff-surgeons, emerging fellows, and house officers. At the core of this educational material is one fundamental principle that guides the methodology—that being to do the right thing for each individual patient in every unique situation.

This book and video series on medical education has greatly expanded on the 2002 publication and includes a great deal of new information on general surgical strategies; the use of protocols including and exceeding those based on the Kidney Dialysis Outcomes Quality Initiative guidelines; the efficacious use of vascular access catheters; a new, broad section on peritoneal dialysis catheters; and an outstanding fourth book presenting a compilation of simulated complex vascular-access challenges with stepwise treatment options and comments by the editors.

This is a very ambitious series dealing with a complex subject. It is a valuable resource for all health care professionals involved in the care of patients with end-stage renal disease or malignancies—for although it is primarily a surgical text, it is a surgical text with a soul; a technical manual with a philosophical message, not simply "First, do no harm," but to "do the right thing."

Robert N. McClelland, M.D., F.A.C.S.
Professor of Surgery
Division of GI/Endocrine Surgery
Founder of ACS Selected Readings in Surgery
Department of Surgery
The University of Texas Southwestern Medical Center at Dallas

INTRODUCTION

The Davidson Medical Series is a comprehensive guide to current common diagnostic, operative, and percutaneous techniques used in creating and maintaining vascular access for dialysis in patients with end-stage renal disease or cancer. When writing the text, the authors have focused on surgeons in training, interventional radiologists, nephrologists and fellows, dialysis nurses, and technicians. Health care professionals involved in the care of patients with end-stage renal disease or cancer and the patients themselves will also benefit from these handbooks. Volumes I through IV are briefly described below.

Volume I, appropriately, covers peritoneal dialysis. The concept of "Peritoneal Dialysis First" states that whenever feasible peritoneal dialysis should be the first dialysis modality considered for patients in need of a lifelong access strategy. Peritoneal dialysis offers a survival benefit for several years after dialysis initiation. Patients who receive a transplant while on peritoneal dialysis have better outcomes compared to patients who are on hemodialysis. As all dialysis access modalities have a high failure rate over time, proactively planning and placing access for hemodialysis in patients on peritoneal dialysis serves as "life insurance," should the peritoneal dialysis modality later fail. Peritoneal dialysis and hemodialysis must not be seen as competitive therapies but rather complementary, where over time both dialysis access options are considered as integral parts of thoughtful long-term planning.

Volume II details the hemodialysis access procedures including wrist radio-cephalic, upper arm brachio-cephalic fistula, the most common vein transposition procedures, and the placement and indications of grafts.

Volume III, in addition to vascular access catheters for dialysis in ESRD, also encompasses the much similar insertion techniques, types and sites used in oncology patients.

Volume IV is a compilation of case reports with color images collected over the past several years. In a "simulated" case-report format, the complex decision making processes for optimum access will be brought into "real life" scenarios facing the dialysis access team. Dialysis aspects that were not included in the first three volumes will find a home in this fourth publication. This volume will include dialysis needle puncture technique, a practical guide on Current Procedural Terminology (CPT) and International Classification of Diseases (ICD-9) coding for dialysis access procedures, common prescription drug administration in dialysis patients, and pre- and post-operative guides for patients and their families.

This series of books and videos reflects the highly technical nature of clinical management of dialysis and oncologic vascular access in an evolving field. This evolution is best illustrated by the rapid, innovative development of interventional radiologic procedures. The series includes instructional photographs and high-definition videos detailing current surgical techniques—because in the medical field, pictures often speak louder than words. With more than 450,000 patients on dialysis in the USA and about 90,000 new patients added every year, surgical vascular access procedures have become the most common procedure in hospitals, not to mention radiologic diagnostic and therapeutic interventions, catheter placements, and dialysis needle punctures for the dialysis treatment itself. Therefore, this educational series also reaches out to dialysis RNs and technologists, with the intent to expand knowledge and understanding of each team member's expertise and roles by emphasizing communication skills in the common health care hierarchy model.

Statements regarding technique and choice of equipment are the opinions of the authors. We recognize that many similarly effective alternatives achieve excellent results. These books address examples of common surgical and interventional procedures, but do not cover all conceivable variations. In this regard, these publications represent our very personal and perhaps slightly biased experience with dialysis and oncologic vascular access.

With new print-on-demand technology, updates to these volumes can be more easily incorporated into future editions. We invite your comments and suggestions to solve specific problems. Please fax them to 214.520.8486 or e-mail drd@ingemardavidson.com.

The Editors
Ingemar Davidson, Maurizio Gallieni, Ramesh Saxena

ABBREVIATIONS

AGE	advanced glycation end-product
AVF	arteriovenous fistulae
CAPD	continuous ambulatory peritoneal dialysis
CCPD	continuous cycling peritoneal dialysis
CFPD	continuous flow peritoneal dialysis
CKD	chronic kidney disease
CMS	Center for Medicare and Medicaid Services
D/P	dialysate to plasma
ESRD	end-stage renal disease
GDP	glucose degradation product
HD	hemodialysis
IAP	intra-abdominal pressure
ISPD	International Society for Peritoneal Dialysis
IV	intravenous
K/DOQI	Kidney Dialysis Outcomes and Quality Initiative
LMA	laryngeal mask airway
NIPD	nocturnal intermittent peritoneal dialysis
PD	peritoneal dialysis
PET	peritoneal equilibration test
RRF	residual renal function
RRT	renal replacement therapy
UF	ultrafiltration

THE DIALYSIS ACCESS ALGORITHM

A Patient Centered Decision-Making Algorithm for Peritoneal Dialysis

I. DAVIDSON, M. GALLIENI, R. SAXENA

Controversy surrounds the establishment of proper planning, placement and management (the best practice pattern) of peritoneal dialysis (PD) access. These include the dialysis type and modality selection, timing of access placement and who places the access. The lack of randomized studies and the difficulty of performing studies with multiple confounding factors in the heterogeneous and changing end-stage renal disease (ESRD) population demographics, partly explains the dialysis access conundrum. Also, the rapidly developing and competing technologies, the wide spectrum of the professional experience, as well as bias and socio-economic forces make the dialysis access algorithms multivariate and complex. This introductory chapter describes a dialysis access algorithm approach to the patient needing renal replacement therapy (RRT), considering long-term improved patient outcome as the ultimate objective. The concept of "Peritoneal Dialysis First" is explained and emphasized.

DEFINING THE PROBLEM

The world population is experiencing a growth of ESRD requiring RRT. In the USA alone, there were over 571,000 patients with ESRD in 2009, consuming 8.1% of the Medicare budget and $42.5 billion in total costs (1). With an annual growth of 4%, the ESRD population is projected to grow to 775,000 patients on dialysis in 2020 (1). Currently there are 3 RRT options: renal transplantation, hemodialysis (HD) and PD. While renal transplantation remains the RRT of choice, the proportion of patients with ESRD receiving renal transplants has not changed in the past decade (1). Thus, the majority of patients with ESRD depend upon various dialysis modalities for sustaining life. For patients with chronic kidney disease (CKD) of stage IV (glomerular filtration rate of 15–30 ml/min), the choice of dialysis modality and therefore dialysis access varies greatly among different countries and communities. Indeed, the choice between dialysis modalities is remarkably different. While PD is the prevalent dialysis mode in less than 8% of USA cases, and 11.4 % in Italy, it is the primary mode of dialysis access in many other countries like UK, New Zealand, and Mexico (1). Complex psychosocial and economic factors, pre-ESRD education, patient preference, nephrology and surgery training patterns, as well as skills and bias are examples of the many confounding factors influencing the crucial selection of the best RRT modality for the individual patient (Table 1.1) (2–6). Proper planning is of paramount importance to the timely initiation of RRT, in order to prevent serious uremic complications, avoid the use of dialysis catheters, and improve patient outcome and quality of life in a cost-effective way (7). Planning for RRT must begin in CKD stage IV to allow time for patients and families to understand various treatment options and make judicious decisions, thereby allowing orderly planned initiation of dialysis with an appropriate access (8). Contrary to trends favoring PD, growth of the ESRD population in the USA has been accompanied by decreased utilization of PD, while the HD modality is exceeding 90% of the dialysis population (9, 10). Some studies suggest that this practice pattern contributes to increased morbidity, mortality, and health care costs (11–14). In the wake of low utilization of arteriovenous fistulae (AVF) (1) and the Kidney Dialysis Outcomes and Quality Initiative (K/DOQI) recommendations (15), the Center for Medicare and Medicaid Services (CMS) launched a National Vascular Access Improvement Initiative in 2003 emphasizing a Fistula First approach, to increase the use of AVFs in the HD patient cohort with the goal of exceeding a prevalent rate of at least 40% in patients with chronic HD (16). This stated goal was raised to 66% and as of August 2011, the AVF rate is 59.5% (17). The PD modality was not considered in this assessment.

DOING THE RIGHT THING AT THE RIGHT TIME

In the broadest term, practice patterns correlate to outcomes including patient and technique survival, access outcome, and cost to society at large. Individuals, institutions, governments, and specialty societies may direct and subliminally influence the selection of dialysis modality. The most visible and widespread effort in this regard is the CMS Fistula First National Vascular Access Improvement Initiative (16). Similarly, the International Society for Peritoneal Dialysis (ISPD) is stressing the underutilization of PD modality, especially in the Western societies (18). The selection of dialysis access is of great importance in planning a successful transition to dialysis treatment of patients approaching ESRD. A sound long-term dialysis access is designed to maximize patient quality of life, improve survival, and be cost-effective. (19) Rather than emphasizing the doctrine of 1 modality fitting all, doing the right thing for each patient, each time, is ethically and morally the better model (Table 1.2). The issue is not who places the access but who does it right, every time, to everyone, and everywhere. It should be outcome and patient driven. The decision-making algorithm for 2 similar patients may therefore vary, based on individual circumstances summarized in Table 1.1. Generally, outcomes of AVFs are superior to those of grafts (20). When used as a patient's first access, AVF survival is superior to grafts regarding time

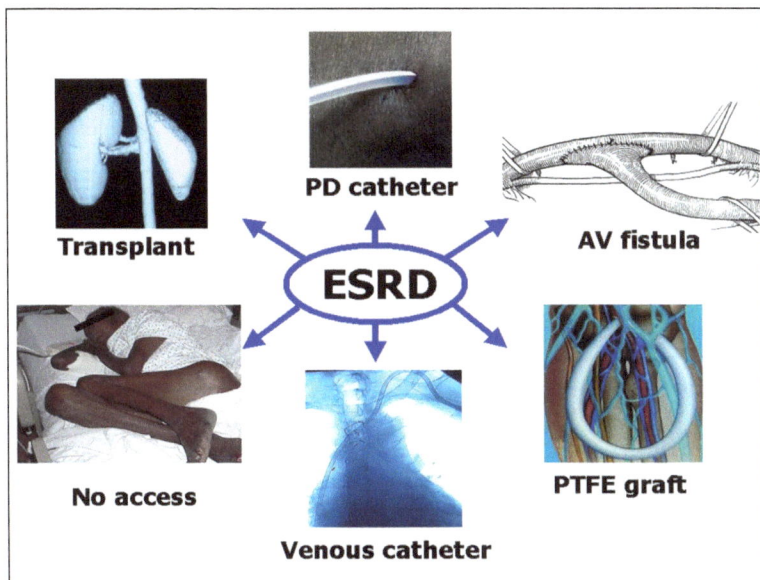

Figure 1.1.   Treatment Options for ESRD from the Perspective of Access Preference Clockwise starting from transplant, 6 treatment options are shown in the approximate order of overall outcome effectiveness. Many confounding forces, some of which are outlined in Table 1.1, influence the decision. During the life of an ESRD patient 3 or even all of these life-sustaining treatments are sequentially or repeatedly used. (Davidson I, Gallieni M, Saxena R, Dolmatch B. A patient centered decision making dialysis access algorithm. *J Vasc Access* 2007; 8: 59–68)

to first failure (RR=0.53) (21). However, no randomized controlled trials have been performed comparing AVFs and grafts, and comparisons may therefore be flawed by a selection bias, since patients with PTFE grafts are older by about 10 years and have higher co-morbidities (diabetes, cardiovascular disease, lupus) associated with poorer vascular anatomy. Although wrist (radiocephalic) and elbow (brachiocephalic) primary AVFs are the preferred HD access type (easy to place, low cost, low complication rate, including lower incidence of infection, and vascular steal phenomenon), they also have drawbacks. The major disadvantage of the wrist (radiocephalic) AVF is a possible lower blood flow rate compared to other access types. Another drawback of radiocephalic AVFs is their initial high failure rate of about 15 % and a secondary patency rate at 1 year of 62% (22). A recent randomized USA multicenter study of 877 AVFs showed non-maturation in excess of 60% (23). In other words, less than 40% of AVFs are used for dialysis at 1 year after placement, sharply contrasting that of 93% for first time placed PD catheters (24). The increasing number of non-matured AVFs has likely resulted in more patients needing long-term catheter dialysis access. The different dialysis modalities and access types must not be seen as competitive, but rather complementary, where the outcome strategy is the effective utilization of RRT treatment options over the patient's lifetime (Figure 1.1).

AN IDEAL WORLD VERSUS REALITY

Figure 1.1 depicts the possible treatment options available to the uremic patient. Three of these alternatives refer to HD: AVFs, PTFE grafts, and central venous catheters. In the ideal world, the impending renal failure diagnosis is proactively managed with a pre-emptive living donor kidney transplant (CKD stage 4–5). In patients with CKD and type I diabetes mellitus, the preferred event is simultaneous kidney and pancreas transplants from a deceased donor. However, a kidney transplant from a living donor followed by a pancreas transplant from a deceased donor is an equally logical option (Figure 1.2). In sharp contrast, because of patient denial and late consideration for dialysis access placement, the reality is plagued by the fact that 80% of all patients initiate HD with a dual-lumen catheter. Moreover, of all current prevalent dialysis patients, only a small fraction (3.7 % or about 15,000) (1) in the USA receives a kidney transplant annually. In situations where timely, accurate, and perhaps passionate pre-ESRD education is given to the patient, a significantly higher number of patients with CKD (40%) choose PD and only a small fraction start HD with a temporary catheter (4–6).

Table 1.1.   Factors Influencing Dialysis Modality Selection
General:
  • Patient desire, including lifestyle, profession
  • Socioeconomic factors
  • Patient education on dialysis issues and options
  • Nephrologists' education (equal education on HD and PD)
  • Comfort level with dialysis modality
  • Co-morbidity severity
  • Surgical experience and technical support
  • Stage of CKD/ESRD
Indications favoring HD:
  • Patient restrictions to learn the PD technique
  • Lack of PD training facilities
  • Abdominal stoma (i.e. colostomy)
  • Recurrent abdominal inflammatory events

Indications favoring PD:
- Veins and arteries unsuitable for HD
- Travel distance to dialysis facility
- Heparin intolerance
- Lower cost than HD

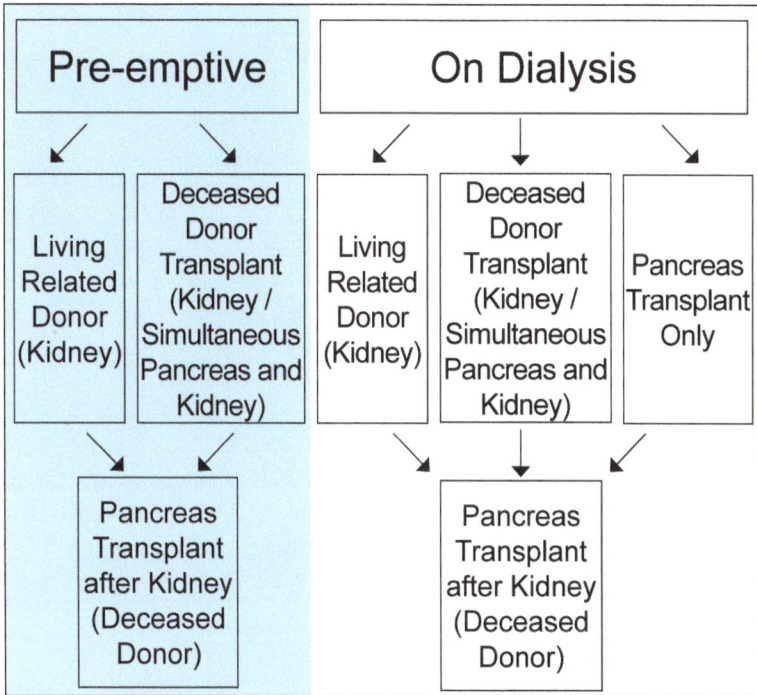

Figure 1.2. ESRD Kidney and Pancreas (type I diabetes only) Transplant Scenarios (Davidson I, Gallieni M, Saxena R, Dolmatch B. A patient centered decision making dialysis access algorithm. *J Vasc Access* 2007; 8: 59–68)

A PRACTICAL PATIENT-DRIVEN ALGORITHM

The following algorithms and strategies outline decision-making processes based on a multitude of factors, some of which are summarized in Table 1.1. The intention is to have universal applications driven by the spirit of the mission statement of *Doing the Right Thing the Right Way*, which is expressed in Table 1.2. This mission statement also implies a seamless and transparent teamwork approach. It represents a continuum-of-care treatment model of the ESRD patient where emphasis is placed on team members being in close geographic proximity (same building) and ideally in the same clinic (25,26). This allows timely decision making between the surgeon, the nephrologists and the interventional radiologist ("one-stop shopping"). This concept also implies fluid, clear, crisp, and effective communication between key team members with emphasis on patient safety, outcome, and comfort. A dialysis access short- and long-term plan should be updated on a regular basis. With a proactive approach, future access problems can be anticipated and addressed with the overall goal to avoid dialysis interruptions, temporary central vein catheters, and associated morbidity.

Philosophically, this approach implies that while striving for the best practice option for each patient, the actual treatment modality may be quite different depending on a complex set of confounding circumstances. For example, the treatment modality option in a large university and research institution will be apart from that seen in a community hospital. The patients' options in a rural area may be limited compared to those in a large western city. Likewise, in many developing countries dialysis and transplantation may not be offered. Also, culture, tradition, and religious beliefs greatly affect the decision making process in treating the ESRD patient.

Table 1.2. A Mission Statement for Your Dialysis Access Team

Do the right thing—

at the right time,

in the right amount,

for the right reason

—within the framework of your conscience,

skills, and knowledge—

modeled by the culture and societal laws

in which you live.

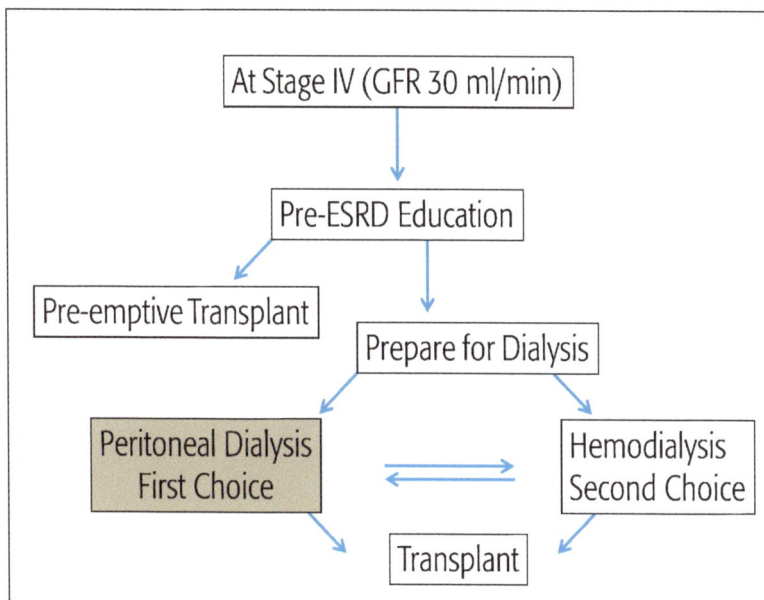

Figure 1.3. ESRD Treatment Modality Algorithm
Although rarely reflected in reality, this diagram depicts a patient driven (optimal) ESRD modality sequential treatment strategy for early detection and progression prevention, emphasizing the benefits of PD as the first option. Abbreviation: GFR, glomerular filtration rate. (Davidson I, Gallieni M, Saxena R, Dolmatch B. A patient centered decision making dialysis access algorithm. *J Vasc Access* 2007; 8: 59–68)

"PERITONEAL DIALYSIS (PD) FIRST, HEMODIALYSIS (HD) SECOND"

The concept of "PD First" implies that whenever feasible PD should be offered as the first dialysis modality (Figure 1.3). First, PD provides a survival benefit for the first several years after dialysis initiation in the majority of patients (27–34). Moreover, patients who receive a transplant while on PD have better long- and short-term transplant outcomes compared to patients who are on HD immediately prior to kidney transplant (35,36). Second, while on PD, plans can be made to place an AVF. The PD option allows extra time for the AVF to mature and for creative access options such as 2-stage surgical procedures to optimize the access outcome effectiveness. As all dialysis access modalities have a high failure rate over time, proactively placing an AVF in a PD patient serves as "life insurance," should the PD modality later fail. The benefits of the PD First concept are summarized in Table 1.3. PD and HD must not be seen as competitive therapies but rather complementary, where over time the dialysis access options are considered as integral parts of thoughtful long-term planning.

Table 1.3. Peritoneal Dialysis Offers Significant Advantages:
- Survival rate on PD better than most patients on HD in first few years of treatment
- Associated with better quality of life
- Patient can remain in the workforce while dialyzing at night
- Greater freedom to travel
- Maintains residual renal function (RRF) longer
- Less early dysfunction after renal transplant
- Better long-term allograft function
- Provides more even/continuous dialysis
- Lower cost
- AVF can be placed and matured, anticipating future HD
- No needle punctures for dialysis
- Fewer blood borne infection transmissions

EARLY REFERRAL AND PRESERVATION OF VEINS

Two seemingly simple measures would dramatically improve the outcomes of future dialysis access. First, early referral to a nephrologist and to an access surgeon for evaluation increases the likelihood for placing an AVF and avoiding morbidity from a temporary catheter (8). Therefore, when GFR approaches 30 ml/min, (CKD stage 4), patient education about RRT and dialysis access must begin with referral for preemptive transplant and dialysis access consideration. Second, preserving veins by preventing venipunctures and intravenous (IV) lines in potential future dialysis access veins for AVF placement also increases the chances for an AVF. Blood draws and IV lines damage potential AVF veins. Only the dorsal aspect of the hand should be allowed for venous blood access. Patients undergoing HD may have blood draws done through their cannulation needles, either at the beginning or at the end of their dialysis treatment, in order to preserve their veins. These are simple policy decisions made by individuals with the vision and mission to do and implement the right thing. Peripherally inserted central catheter (PICC) lines must not be used in patients with future dialysis need, and certainly not in stage 4–5 ESRD patients. Although educational efforts have been made, intense concerted education of hospital workers must take place for both of these measures to become universally applied and consistently effective.

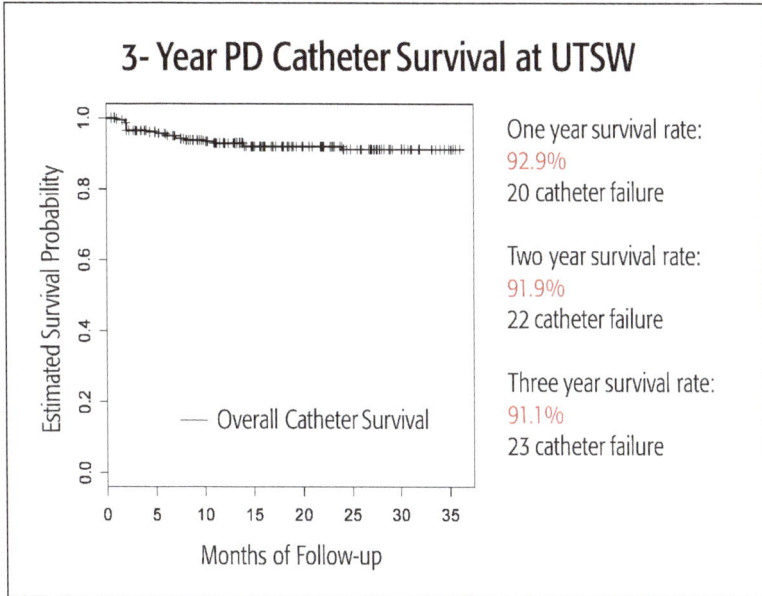

3- Year PD Catheter Survival at UTSW

One year survival rate:
92.9%
20 catheter failure

Two year survival rate:
91.9%
22 catheter failure

Three year survival rate:
91.1%
23 catheter failure

— Overall Catheter Survival

Estimated Survival Probability

Months of Follow-up

Figure 1.4. Three-Year PD Catheter Survival at UT Southwestern Medical Center
The 1-, 2-, and 3-year first-time placement PD catheter survival rates were 92.9%, 91.9%. and 91.1%, respectively, representing the most optimal dialysis modality in properly selected patients. (Singh N, Davidson I, Minhajuddin A, et al. Risk factors associated with peritoneal dialysis catheters survival: A nine year single center study in 315 patients. *J Vasc Access* 2010; 11: 316.)

CENTRAL VEIN DIALYSIS CATHETERS

Due to lack of permanent access—often caused by late referral and patient denial—an astounding 80% of patients start dialysis with a temporary central-vein catheter. While the use of central-vein HD catheters is often life saving, there is a remarkable variation between 2–40% in their indications and frequency between dialysis units. Of all prevalent patients on HD in the USA (37) 6.6% were using a catheter while awaiting AVF maturation. This number doubled in 2 years from 3.8% in Oct 2003. The national prevalent average catheter use in the USA was 27.0 % in 2005—in contrast, the K/DOQI guidelines aim for less than 10%. (15). It will take concentrated educational efforts of the dialysis unit personnel, surgeons, nephrologists, radiologists, and the patients in order to reduce central-vein catheter utilization. These efforts for improvement initiatives in dialysis access in general are urgently needed. Organizational and fiscal support currently is not well defined.

STRATEGIES FOR SAFE AND TIMELY INITIATION OF FLUID EXCHANGES AFTER PLACEMENT OF A CATHETER

The policy in most PD units recommends waiting 3–4 weeks before fluid exchanges. In case of an urgent need for dialysis, a PD treatment may be started with small-volume exchanges (i.e. 1000–1500 ml), rather than placing a central-vein catheter (38,39). If small umbilical, incisional, or inguinal hernias are repaired with mesh, without entering the peritoneal cavity, dialysis can continue without delay. In other cases, small-volume exchanges for 2–4 weeks may be appropriate. After an open laparotomy procedure or other extensive procedures, a temporary internal jugular catheter for 3–4 weeks is indicated.

SUMMARY

A detailed review of patient history and a patient examination are the mainstay of dialysis access modality selection, including site and type of access. Regular patient examinations and careful maintenance of the vascular access site increase longevity. As a lifelong access strategy, PD should be considered as the first dialysis modality in all suitable cases. Once initiated, PD care should include appropriate planning for eventual HD access.

REFERENCES

1. United States Renal Data System, *Annual Data Report* 2009. www.usrd.org
2. Stack AG. Determinants of modality selection among incident dialysis patients: Results from a national study. *J Am Soc Nephrol* 2002; 13: 1279–87.
3. Mehrotra R, Blake P, Berman N, Nolph KD. An analysis of dialysis training in the United States and Canada. *Am J Kidney Dis* 2002; 40: 152–60.
4. Golper T. Patient education: can it maximize the success of therapy? *Nephrol Dial Transplant* 2001; 16 (suppl 7): S20–4.
5. Jager KJ, Korevaar JC, Dekker FW, et al. The effect of contraindications and patient preference on dialysis modality selection in ESRD patients in the Netherlands. *Am J Kidney Dis* 2004; 43: 891–9.
6. Korevaar JC, Boeschoten EW, Dekker FW, et al. What have we learned about PD from recent major clinical trials? *Perit Dial Int* 2007; 27: 11–5.

7.   Levin A, Lewis M, Mortiboy P, et al. Multidisciplinary predialysis programs. Quantifica-
     tion and limitations of their impact on patient outcomes in two Canadian settings. *Am J
     Kidney Dis* 1997, 29: 533–40.

8.   National Kidney Foundation. K/DOQI clinical practice guidelines for chronic kidney
     disease: Evaluation, classification and stratification. Kidney Disease Outcome Quality
     Initiative. *Am J Kidney Dis* 2002; 39 (suppl): S1–246.

9.   Kaufman JL. The decline of autogenous hemodialysis access site. *Semin Dial* 1995; 8: 59–
     61.

10. The cost effectiveness of alternate types of vascular access and the economics cost of
     ESRD. Bethesda MD. *National Institute of Diabetes and Digestive and Kidney Diseases* 1995;
     139–57.

11. Xue JL, Dahl D, Ebben JP, et al. The association of initial hemodialysis access type with
     mortality outcomes in elderly Medicare ESRD patients. *Am J Kidney Dis* 2003; 42: 1013–9.

12. Polkinghorne KR, McDonald SP, Atkins RC, et al. Vascular access and all cause mortality.
     A propensity score analysis. *J Am Soc Nephrol* 2004; 15: 477–86.

13. Kinchen KS, Sadler J, Fink N, et al. The timing of specialist evaluation in chronic kidney
     disease and mortality. *Ann Intern Med* 2002; 137: 479–48.

14. Stack AG. Impact of timing of nephrology referral and pre-ESRD care on mortality risk
     among new ESRD patients in the United States. *Am J Kidney Dis* 2003, 41: 310–8.

15. National Kidney Foundation. K/DOQI clinical practice guidelines for vascular access up-
     date 2006. *Am J Kidney Dis* 2006; 48 (suppl 1): S176–S322.

16. National Vascular Access Improvement Project. CMS launches "Fistula First" initiative
     to improve care and quality of life for hemodialysis patients. Press release April 14, 2004.
     http://www.cms.hhs.gov/aaps/media/press/release.asp?counter=1007.

17. Fistula First Breakthrough. 2004. http://www.cms.gov/ESRDQualityImproveInit/04_
     FistulaFirstBreakthrough.asp.

18. Blake PG. Peritoneal dialysis in the USA. *Perit Dial Int* 2006; 26: 416–8.

19. Arora P, Kausz AT, Obrador GT, et al. Hospital utilization among chronic dialysis patients.
     J Am Soc Nephrol 2000; 11: 740–6.

20. NKF-K/DOQI Clinical Practice Guidelines for Vascular Access. *Am J Kidney Dis* 2006; 48
     (suppl 1): S176–S322.

21. Pisoni RL, Young EW, Dykstra DM, et al. Vascular access use in Europe and the United
     States: Results from the DOPPS. *Kidney Int* 2002; 61: 305–16.

22. Rooijens PP, Tordoir JH, Stijnen T, Burgmans JP, Smet de AA, Yo TI. Radiocephalic wrist
     arteriovenous fistula for hemodialysis: Meta-analysis indicates a high primary failure
     rate. *Eur J Vasc Endovasc Surg* 2004; 28: 583–9.

23. Dember LM, Beck GJ, Allon M, et al, for the Dialysis Access Consortium Study Group. Ef-
     fect of Clopidogrel on early failure of arteriovenous fistulas for hemodialysis. A random-
     ized control trial. *JAMA*. 2008; 299: 2164–2171.

24. Singh N, Davidson I, Minhajuddin A, et al. Risk factors associated with peritoneal dialysis
     catheters survival: A nine year single center study in 315 patients. *J Vasc Access* 2010; 11:
     316.

25. Davidson IJA, Gallieni M, Saxena R. Our algorithm for determining the best dialysis access. *J Vasc Access* 2006; 7: 143–6.

26. Davidson IJA. Access clinic, access decisions and multi-disciplinary care our patients deserve. *J Vasc Access* 2006; 7: 235–8.

27. Collins AJ, Hao W, Xia H, et al. Mortality risks of peritoneal dialysis and hemodialysis. *Am J Kidney Dis* 1999; 34: 1065–74.

28. Fenton SSA, Schaubel DE, Desmeules M, et al. Hemodialysis versus peritoneal dialysis: A comparison of adjusted mortality rates. *Am J Kidney Dis* 1997; 30:334–42.

29. Korevaar JC, Feith GW, Dekker FW, et al. Effect of starting with hemodialysis compared with peritoneal dialysis in patients new on dialysis treatment: A randomized controlled trial. *Kidney Int* 2003; 64: 2222–8.

30. Vonesh EF, Snyder JJ, Foley RN, Collins AJ. The differential impact of risk factors on mortality in hemodialysis and peritoneal dialysis. *Kidney Int* 2004; 66: 2389–401.

31. Termorshuizen F, Korevaar JC, Dekker FW, Van Manen JG, Boeschoten EW, Krediet RT. Hemodialysis and peritoneal dialysis: Comparison of adjusted mortality rates according to the duration of dialysis: Analysis of the Netherlands cooperative study on adequacy of dialysis. *J Am Soc Nephrol* 2003; 14: 2851–60.

32. Jaar BG, Coresh J, Plantinga IC, et al. Comparing the risk for death with peritoneal dialysis and hemodialysis in a national cohort of patients with chronic kidney disease. *Ann Int Med* 2005; 143: 174–83.

33. Ganesh SK, Hulbert-Shearon T, Port FK, Eagle K, Stack A. Mortality differences by dialysis modality among incident ESRD patients with and without coronary artery disease. *J Am Soc Nephrol* 2003; 14: 415–24.

34. Stack AG, Molony DA, Rahman NS, Dosekun A, Murthy . Impact of dialysis modality on survival of new ESRD patients with congestive heart failure in the United States. *Kidney Int* 2003; 64: 1071–9.

35. Bleyer AJ, Burkart JM, Russell GB, Adams PL. Dialysis modality and delayed graft function after cadaveric renal transplantation. *J Am Soc Nephrol* 1999; 10:154–9.

36. Goldfarb-Rumyanitzev AS, Hundle JF, Scandling JD, Baird BC, Cheung AK. The role of pre-transplantation renal replacement therapy modality in kidney allograft and recipient survival. *Am J Kidney Dis* 2005; 46: 537–49.

37. Center for Medicare & Medicaid Services: 2004 Annual Report. End Stage Renal Disease Clinical Performance Measures Project. Baltimore, MD, Department of Health and Human Services, Center for Medicare & Medicaid Services, Center for Beneficiary Services, 2004.

38. Gokal R, Alexander S, Ash S, et al. Peritoneal catheters and exit site practices toward optimum peritoneal access:1998 update. *Perit Dial Int* 1998; 18: 11–33.

39. Pirano B, Bailie GR, Bernardini J, et al. Peritoneal dialysis-related infections recommendations: 2005 update. *Perit Dial Int* 2005; 25: 107–31.

OPEN SURGICAL PLACEMENT OF A TWO CUFF, COILED CATHETER

I. DAVIDSON, A. PARAMESH, E. PEDEN, D. SLAKEY

The detailed operative procedures described below are summarized in Chapter 3, which also includes surgical safety and instruments checklists. Videos have also been produced for viewing the open and laparoscopic PD catheter placement techniques described in Chapters 2, 3, and 4.

PLANNING THE SURGERY

■ 1. Choose a catheter for the patient. The different catheters—types, lengths, number of cuffs, and manufacturers—are detailed in Chapter 5. The authors prefer a catheter with a straight neck, 2 cuffs, and a coiled intra-abdominal segment (Figure 2.1). The basic choices include:

One or Two Cuffs? The 2-cuff catheter is preferred as it provides an additional barrier from bacterial migration along the catheter tract (1–3). The subcutaneous cuff is placed 1.5–2.0 cm away from the skin exit site, which keeps the catheter from sliding in and out. Sliding of the catheter at the exit site, as is the case with only 1 cuff, likely induces catheter tract infection. Retrospective reviews suggest double-cuff configurations have a longer catheter survival time, delayed first episode of peritonitis (1–3), as well as a trend towards decreased episodes of peritonitis (4). A second cuff, placed outside the peritoneum membrane, is usually sutured to the posterior rectus fascia in the open procedure as described below in this chapter. With the laparoscopic technique, the cuff is usually lodged in the rectus muscle tissue. This cuff is referred to as the peritoneal cuff throughout this publication. The peritoneal cuff must never be placed inside the abdominal cavity.

Straight or Coiled Intra-Abdominal Segment? Catheters with a coiled intra-abdominal segment are preferred perhaps with the exception of the self-locating (Di Paolo) straight catheter (Figure 5.13) (5). Coiled catheters have about 60 holes along the sides of the coiled portion of the tubing, facilitating the passage of fluid in and out of the abdominal cavity, compared to half that number in the straight configuration. A coiled catheter is heavier than the shorter, straight catheters and therefore tends to stay in the lower pelvis by gravity. The straight, self-locating (Di Paolo) catheter includes a weight at the distal end to stabilize its location in the pelvis. Coiled catheters come in left- and right-side configurations—a choice dictated by the side of the body in which the catheter will be placed. The only difference between the two is the orientation of the radiopaque line on the catheter. This line provides easy x-ray visualization of the catheter course, and may be useful in identifying possible kinks in the catheter.

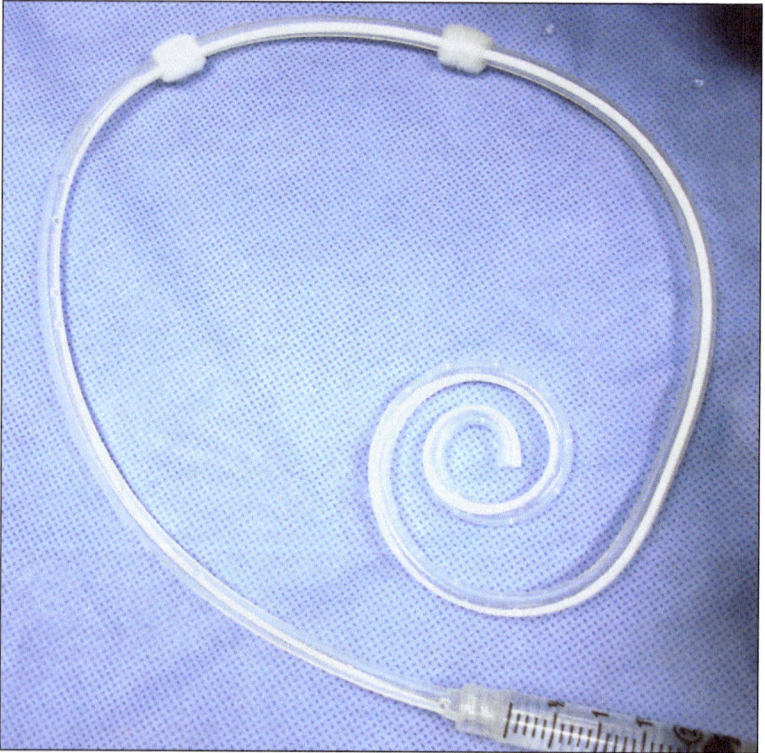

Figure 2.1. Tenckhoff Catheter, 2 Cuffs, Straight Neck, Coiled Intra-abdominal Segment
A syringe is connected to the catheter (visible in the lower right corner).

Straight (flexible) Neck or Preformed Curved Neck (Swan Neck)? A catheter with a preformed bend between the cuffs (Swan Neck) is designed to prevent the coiled portion from migrating upward or side-to-side in the patient's abdomen. Though the feature is beneficial, a catheter with a preformed bend limits the surgeon's flexibility in determining the optimum path for the subcutaneous catheter tubing. With a straight (flexible) neck, the surgeon can tailor the subcutaneous path for each patient's unique anatomy; the 2 cuffs hold the tubing in its arched path. A properly placed arch between the 2 cuffs of a catheter with a straight (flexible) neck provides functionality equal to that of a catheter with a preformed bend.

■ 2. Determine the optimum location for the catheter and mark the skin.

Ideally, the coiled portion of the PD catheter is located in the true pelvis, allowing for proper dialysate instillation and removal/exchanges. This is achieved by choosing the appropriate catheter length, followed by precise placement of the incision/exit site (Figure 2.2). For most adults, the 62.5 cm 2-cuff catheter is the appropriate length; as some adjustment to length can be made with the positioning of cuffs and the peritoneal and skin exit sites. The skin exit site must be easily accessible, visible for the patient, away from the beltline, skin folds, and scars. The subcutaneous tunnel should be fashioned to avoid catheter stresses and kinks. A history of prior non-inflammatory, open abdominal operations does not preclude PD placement (6,7).

Preoperative evaluation includes careful consideration of incision and catheter exit site. Thoughts must be given to the patient's general wishes, body habitus, and possible future transplant incision sites. Most patients are scared. Listen carefully to questions. Your nurse coordinator is more likely to relate to the patient's and family's concerns. Each patient deserves careful evaluation and to be fully informed about surgery, the options, and likely outcome.

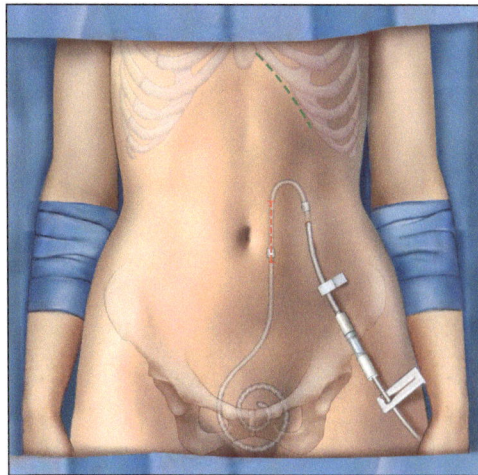

Figure 2.2. Surgical Anatomy in Relation to Open Catheter Placement
PD catheter placement depicting a para-umbilical transrectus muscle approach. The coiled intra-abdominal segment of the catheter is positioned in the pelvic area, with the upper part of the curl at the level of the pubic bone.

General considerations for determining the location for the catheter
- Avoid the beltline area for placement of the exit site.
- Avoid skin folds or previous surgical incision scars as moisture around the exit site predisposes for infection.
- Avoid the side where a future kidney transplant incision might be made.

In a virgin abdomen, the left side is chosen for PD catheter insertion, since the right iliac fossa is the preferred site for a first kidney transplant. The left side may also be advantageous as the intestinal peristalsis movements are directed downward while upward motions predominate in the right side of the abdomen.

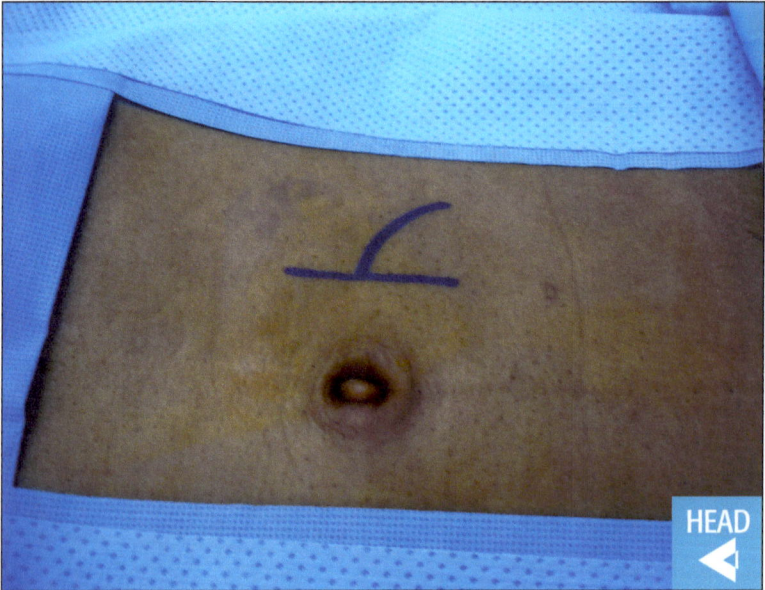

Figure 2.3. Preoperative Marking of the Skin Incision and Exit Site
In this virgin abdomen, the catheter is placed away from the beltline on the left side to facilitate a future kidney transplant on the right side.

People wear their belts at different levels. The patient in Figure 2.4 wears his belt above the umbilicus. However, many have their belt low, perhaps below a protruding abdomen or just above the hipbone. It is important to mark the exit site before surgery with the patient standing. The most common site is depicted in Figures 2.3 and 2.4.

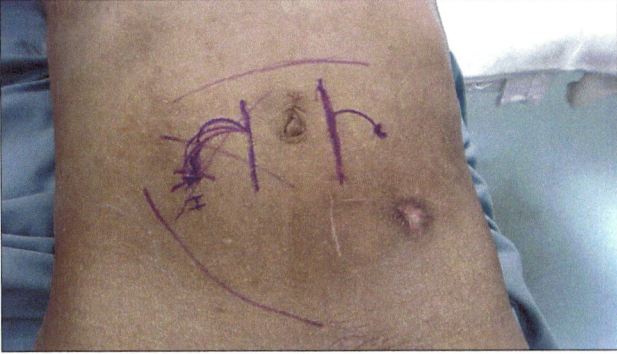

Figure 2.4. Surgical Marks Revised before Surgery
This is an example of a change in pre-operative marking for placement of
the catheter. The original marking on the patient's right side was struck
through and remarked on the left side. An exit site on the right side would
likely result in a future kidney transplant being placed on the left side,
which is technically somewhat harder for anatomical reasons.

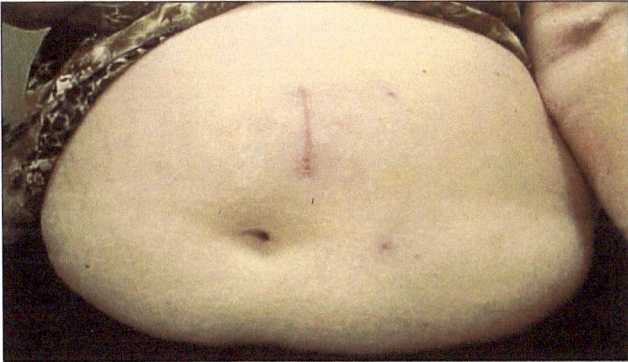

Figure 2.5. An Incision Placed Too High, Causing Omentum Entrapment
of the Catheter

It is wise to reassess the patient and mark the skin on the day of surgery.
In the case depicted in Figure 2.4, the house officer (without checking the at-
tending clinician's notes and a hand drawn picture) had erroneously marked
the right side for PD catheter placement. The marks are redrawn on the left
side, to allow for a future kidney transplant on the right. The scar on the left
lower abdomen is from a laparoscopically placed PD catheter, which was
placed too low, and ended up in the right iliac fossa and tangled up in omental
tissue.

PD catheter placement in obese individuals requires special consideration. In recent years, even morbid obesity is not a contraindication to PD. The image in Figure 2.5 illustrates a common mistake— placing the catheter too high, where the coiled portion will not quite reach the pelvis, resulting in omental entrapment requiring revision. Figure 2.6 depicts the catheter incision and exits site on an overweight individual. PD catheters in obese patients work surprisingly well and are not associated with lower catheter survival rates (6).

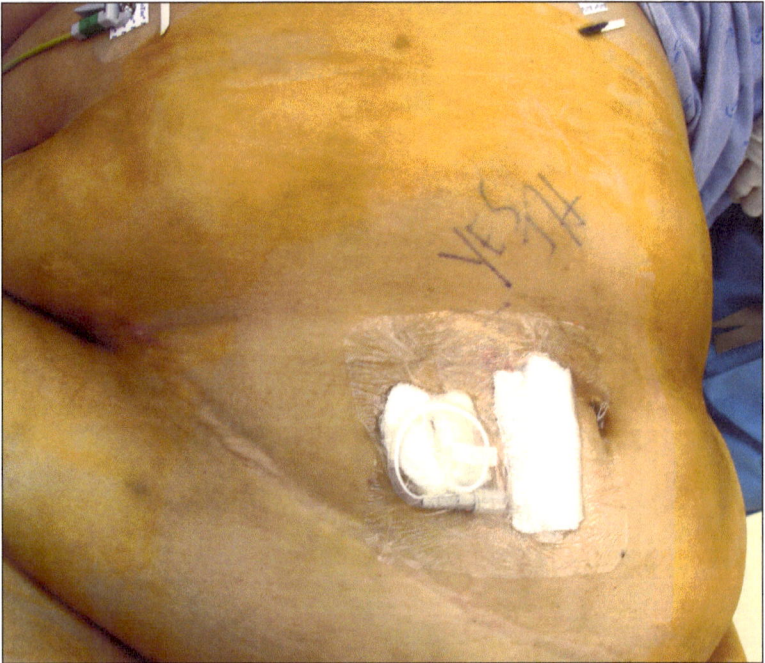

Figure 2.6. Patient Immediately after PD Catheter Placement
The incision is made at the level of the umbilicus, which (unlike the patient in Figure 2.5) is low enough for the coiled section to reach and rest in the pelvic area. This patient had a previous transplant (as seen from the scar in the lower-right abdomen); therefore, the catheter is placed on the right side to avoid interfering with a possible kidney transplant incision on the left side.

It is important to make sure that you and your patient agree on the catheter exit site. Marking the skin for surgery takes place 3 times.

1. In the clinic or surgeon's office, with the patient's involvement, prior to scheduling surgery.
2. In the hospital's preoperative area, on the day of surgery, with the patient's involvement. This provides an opportunity to consider things that may have changed since the office visit, or to answer additional questions.
3. In the operating room, with the surgical team members.

Clearly mark, with an indelible pen (Figure 2.7), the incision as well as the intended subcutaneous tract and exit site of the catheter (Figure 2.3 and 2.4) Having the patient stand is especially important in cases where there is abundant abdominal fat that changes position as the body moves.

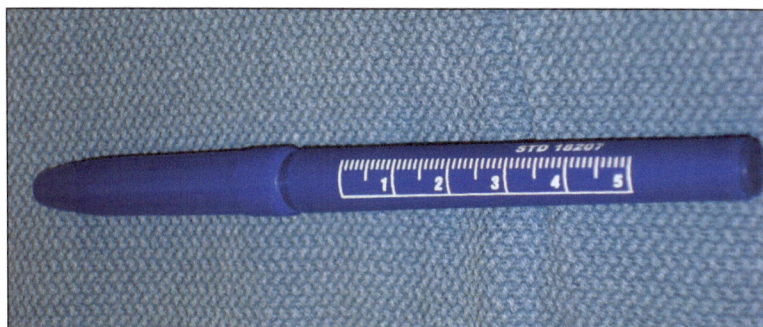

Figure 2.7. Indelible Marking Pen
The marking pen is a powerful tool that may prevent unnecessary errors while providing the surgical team with a clear concept of the operation.

3. Choose a subcutaneous tunneler (The Faller Tunneler or the #15 Blake Drain) for making the subcutaneous exit path.

    The choice of tunneler depends on the location, length, and shape of the subcutaneous exit path, which varies from patient to patient. The diameters of the Faller and #15 Blake drain (Figure 2.8) are the same as the diameter of the catheter. A snug fit between the tube and the skin prevents migration of the subcutaneous cuff without the need for stitches at the exit site.

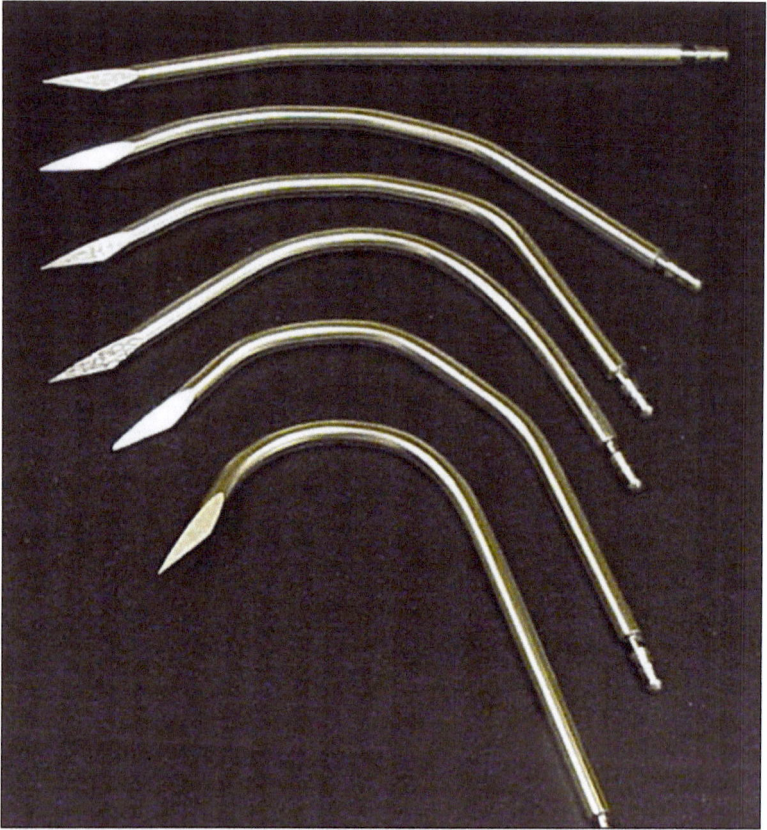

Figure 2.8. A Selection of Blake Drain Trocars
A trocar is used to make a subcutaneous tunnel through the tissues and pierce through
the skin at the exit site. Tunnelers are designed with various bends to fit different needs.
The author most commonly uses the trocar displayed in the bottom of this figure, shown
again in Figure 2.30.

PREOPERATIVE STEPS
Steps performed in the hospital's preoperative area.

1. With the patient's involvement, review the location for the catheter and
   the incision marks made previously.

2. Give the antibiotics—Cefazolin, 1 gram IV piggyback. In cases of allergy: Vancomycin 500 –1000 mg, Clindamycin 600 mg, or Levofloxacin

500 mg IV are alternative options for adults. In cases where it is not practical to give the antibiotics in the preoperative area, they can be given in the operating room before the skin incision.

OPERATIVE STEPS

The para-umbilical open placement of a PD catheter is the author's preferred open technique and is described in detail in the following steps.

General Notes about Open versus Laparoscopic Placement

Peritoneal dialysis catheters are typically inserted using either an open approach or a laparoscopic technique, dictated by the level of comfort of the operating surgeon, the patient's medical risk, and institutional resources. PD catheter placement using the blind Seldinger technique, under fluoroscopic guidance, and or under peritoneoscopic visualization are strongly discouraged because of increased risk of inadvertent visceral injury (8).

The open approach is associated with a shorter operating time and can be performed under spinal or local anesthesia, although general anesthesia is preferred (3,9,10–16). Laparoscopic placement usually requires general anesthesia, which may preclude some patients from undergoing placement. The laparoscopic approach makes it possible to perform additional indicated procedures under direct visualization including placement of the tip of the catheter and securing the tip of the catheter in the pelvis (13,15), as well as the ability to repair umbilical hernias with lysis of adhesions, and omentopexy (10,16). The open approach is more cost-effective, as only basic equipment is required for the procedure (17). Laparoscopy is the best technique to rescue problem catheters (10,18). Comparisons of open versus laparoscopic PD placement do not favor one technique over another (14,15). A thorough evaluation of the patient's suitability for PD, followed with mindful, patient-driven decisions and doing the *right* thing each time is likely to yield the overall best outcome for each patient. (Table 1.2)

The open technique of PD catheter placement is discussed in detail in this chapter and summarized in checklist format in Chapter 3. The laparoscopic technique is detailed in Chapter 4.

General Notes about Anesthesia

Many patients undergoing dialysis access have uremic symptoms, with significant co-morbidity, most notably heart disease, hypertension, anemia, and diabetes. Dosing of anesthesia drugs must be decreased accordingly and given with great caution to avoid serious complications including intra-operative respiratory and circulatory arrest, hypotension—not only jeopardizing the procedure itself but also inducing other complications such as strokes, cardiac events, or requirements for intubations and prolonged ventilator treatment. Although PD catheter placement can be performed under local anesthesia, including epidural with sedation, most PD catheter placements should be carried out under general anesthesia with a safe airway. HIV and Hepatitis C positive individuals are candidates for epidural or general anesthesia to protect the operating room personnel from sudden movement in a sedated patient having a less than optimal regional block. Likewise, laparoscopic placement of PD catheters is done under general anesthesia with endotracheal intubation (Figure 2.9). A laryngeal mask airway (LMA) may not represent a safe airway when changing the patient's position on the operating table is part of the procedure. Supplemental local anesthesia 0.25−0.5 % bupivacaine (Marcaine) in all dialysis access surgery induces a postoperative pain-free period of up to 12 hours, allowing the patient to reach home before needing additional oral pain medication.

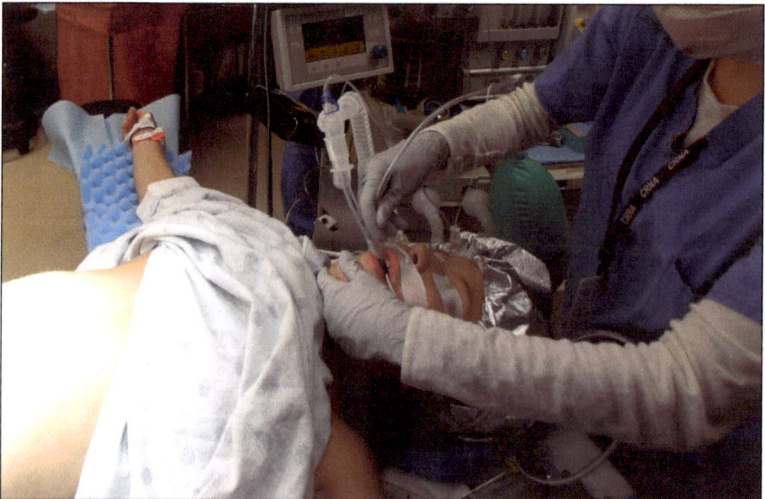

Figure 2.9. General Anesthesia with Endotracheal Intubation is Preferred

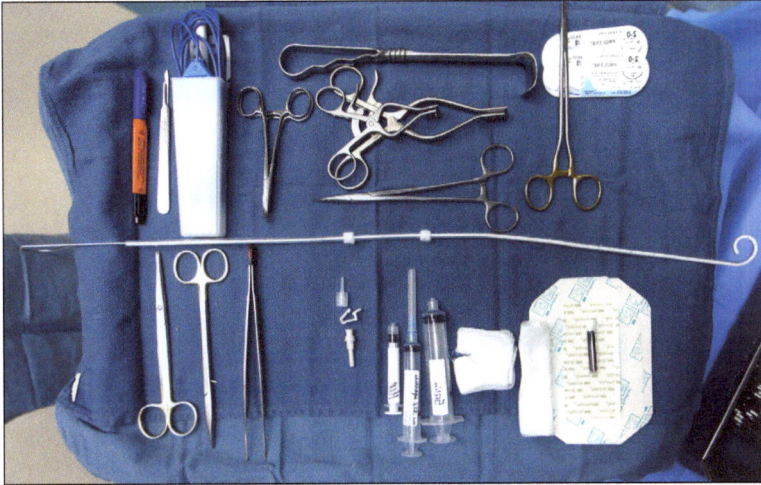

Figure 2.10. The Basic Operating Room PD Instrument Tray

This operating room instrument tray for open placement of the 2-cuff PD catheter is an example of the author's approach to a consistent, efficient and safe working environment, where instruments are kept in the same place at all times and in the order of initial anticipated use. (This concept is consistent with what a commercial airline pilot expects and will indeed find every time he or she walks into the airplane cockpit.)

1. The surgical team pauses to verify the patient's name, medical record number or identification number, surgical side (right or left), incision site, and type of procedure. The surgeon briefs the team of any anticipated procedural deviations. Instruments and supplies are logged and checked into the operating room on the Instruments Checklist. Items listed on the Safety Checklists are checked off (Does the patient have allergies? Have antibiotics been given?).

2. Prepare the abdomen for surgery—shave as needed, prep, and drape.

3. Remark the skin with a sterile, indelible marking pen. The skin incision and exit site are remarked, as needed, to make visible any marks that may have faded since the last marking.

4. Incise the skin with a #15 blade, approximately 3 cm from the umbilicus (Figures 2.2 and 2.3).

■ 5. Carry the dissection down through the subcutaneous tissue to the anterior rectus muscle fascia, using a # 15 blade and/or electrocautery (setting: 20–25), maintaining exact hemostasis.

■ 6. Incise the anterior rectus muscle fascia longitudinally with fine scissors or electrocautery. Split the rectus muscle layers bluntly down to the posterior rectus fascia (Figure 2.11). Electrocauterize, tie, or clip the intra-rectus muscle vessels as appropriate. The posterior fascia is exposed. Exposure is improved by using a Wheitlaner retractor (Figure 2.11) or handheld Senn or US Army retractors (Figure 2.12) as mandated by the case-specific surgical anatomy to optimize exposure.

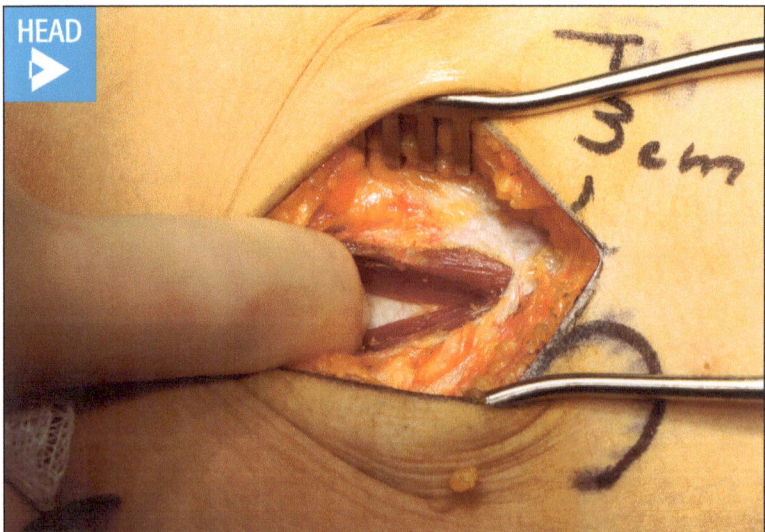

Figure 2.11. Rectus Muscle Gently Split Using an Index Finger

■ 7. Place 1 or 2 tonsil (or Mosquito) hemostats to lift the fascia (and peritoneum) up and away from the intra-abdominal contents. Using fine scissors, incise a small hole (3 mm) through the posterior rectus fascia and the peritoneum, only large enough to facilitate insertion of the PD catheter (Figures 2.12–2.15). The small bowel may be adhered to the anterior abdominal wall, so great care must be taken to protect the small bowel from accidental entry or clipping. Make absolutely certain that free abdominal cavity is present by gently probing with a blunt instrument through the small incision. This is of even greater significance in cases with previous abdominal operations.

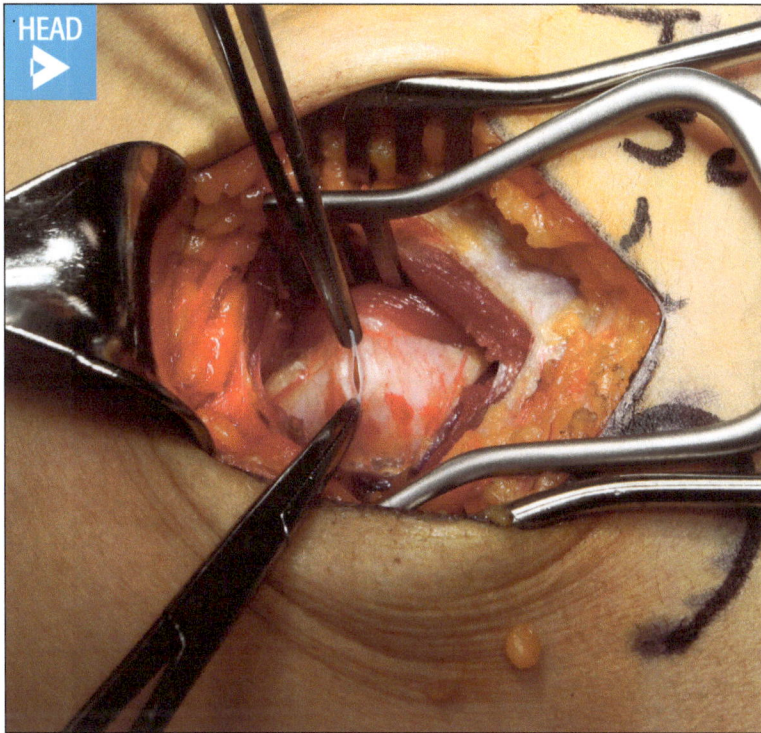

Figure 2.12. A Small Incision Made Through the Posterior Rectus Muscle Fascia and the Peritoneum (Step 7)

In thin individuals, these 2 structures may appear as one. In obese patients various amounts of tissue fills the space between the posterior rectus fascia and peritoneum. Great care is taken not to mistake the small bowel for the peritoneum.

8. Using a size 2-0 non-absorbable polypropylene suture with a 1/2 circle, taper point, 26 mm needle (Prolene Suture, 2-0, SH needle; Ethicon/USA), make a purse-string suture (Figure 2.13) by taking several (6–8) fairly small and tightly-spaced stitches 5 mm away from and around the small hole, stitching through the posterior rectus fascia and the peritoneum. To prevent the accidental suturing of intra-abdominal structures, lift the peritoneum with a blunt instrument (such as a curved or right angle hemostat). Tie the suture behind and cephalad of the cuff (Figures 2.14 and 2.15). Placing the tie in this manner positions it so that ends of the purse-string suture can later be: a) tied around the catheter making a "watertight" seal (Step 11) (Figure 2.23) and, b) sewed to the posterior aspect of the peritoneal Dacron cuff (Step 12) (Figure 2.24).

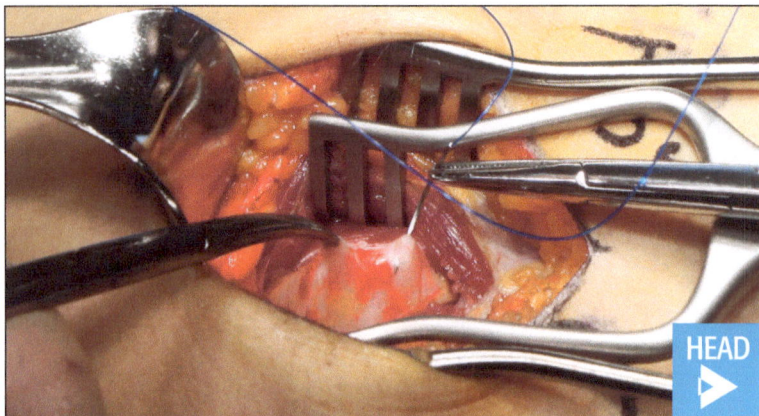

Figure 2.13. Purse-string Suture

Several sutures (6–8), placed about 5 mm away from and around the small peritoneum hole, complete the purse-string using a permanent suture such as a size 2-0 Prolene Suture on a SH needle. A curved hemostat may be inserted to lift the peritoneum to prevent accidental suturing of intra-abdominal structures.

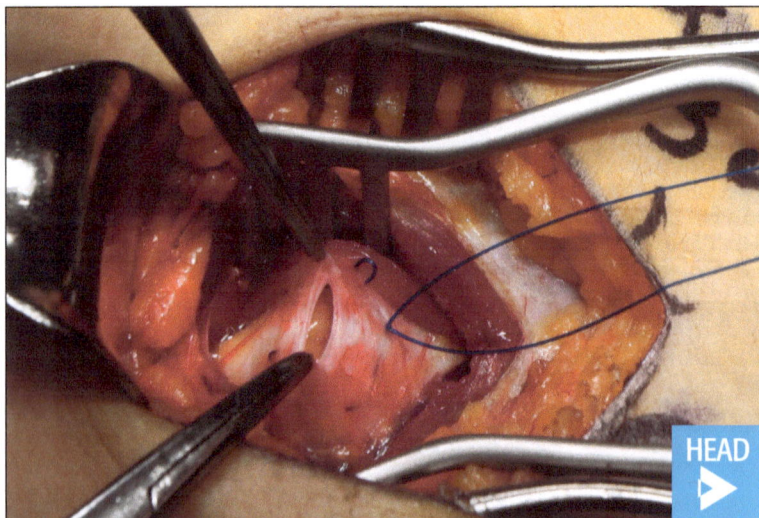

Figure 2.14. Completed Prolene Suture via Purse-string Technique

Steps 1 through 8 have been completed in this image. Several sutures (6–8), placed about 5 mm away from and around the small peritoneum hole, complete the purse-string. A curved hemostat is inserted into the hole to lift the peritoneum and prevent accidental suturing of intra-abdominal structures.

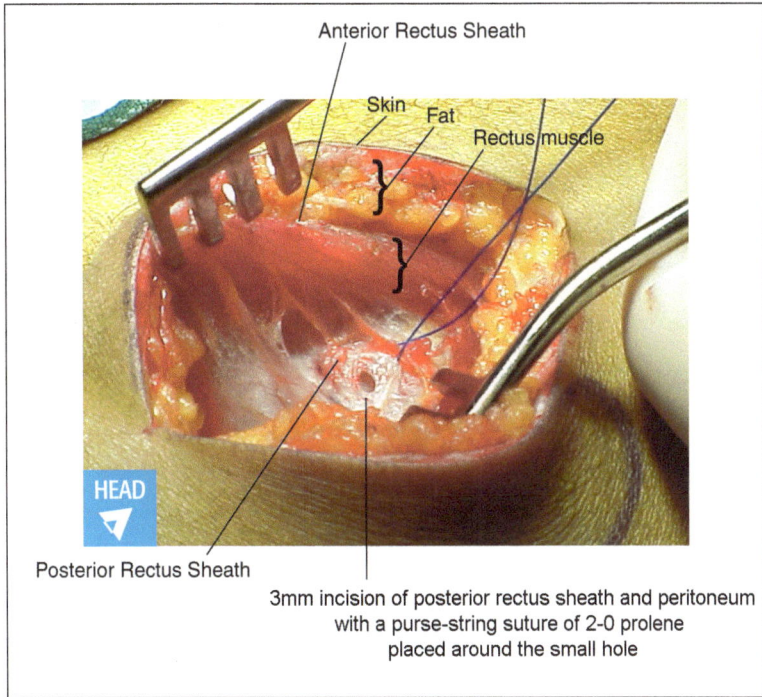

Figure 2.15. Surgical Anatomy and Exposure during PD Catheter Placement
Steps 1–9 have been completed in this image.

9. The intra-abdominal catheter placement is facilitated by using a stiff-ening stylet (Figure 2.16) inserted into the catheter to straighten the curved neck (Figure 2.17) and the coiled intra-abdominal segment (Figure 2.18). Straightening the catheter makes insertion through the small peritoneum opening easy and atraumatic. The tip of the stiff sty-let must not pass outside the (straightened) coiled end to avoid visceral injuries when the catheter is inserted into the body (Figure 2.19).

In order for the stylet to slide into the catheter, the catheter must be filled with saline. In addition, wet gauze around the stylet as it enters the catheter further facilitates easy gliding. (Figure 2.20) The stylet will not slide against a dry surface, which is most important when the stiff stylet is being pulled out. A small amount of surgical lubrication makes the stylet slide with great ease. Figure 2.21 shows the stylet fully inserted into the catheter.

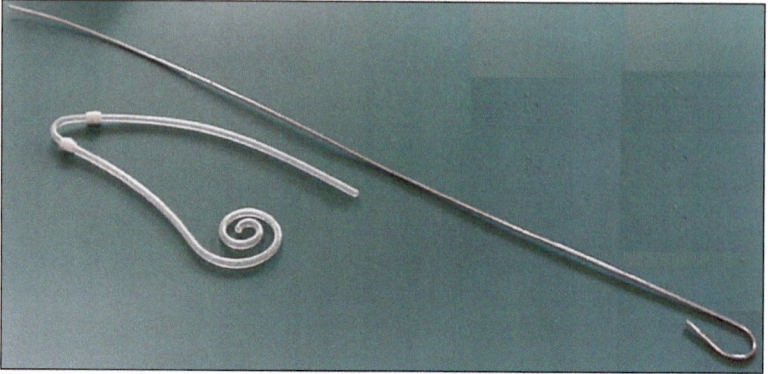

Figure 2.16. Catheter and Stiffening Stylet
The stiffening stylet will be inserted into the catheter to straighten the curved neck and coiled portions, facilitating the insertion through the small peritoneal incision.

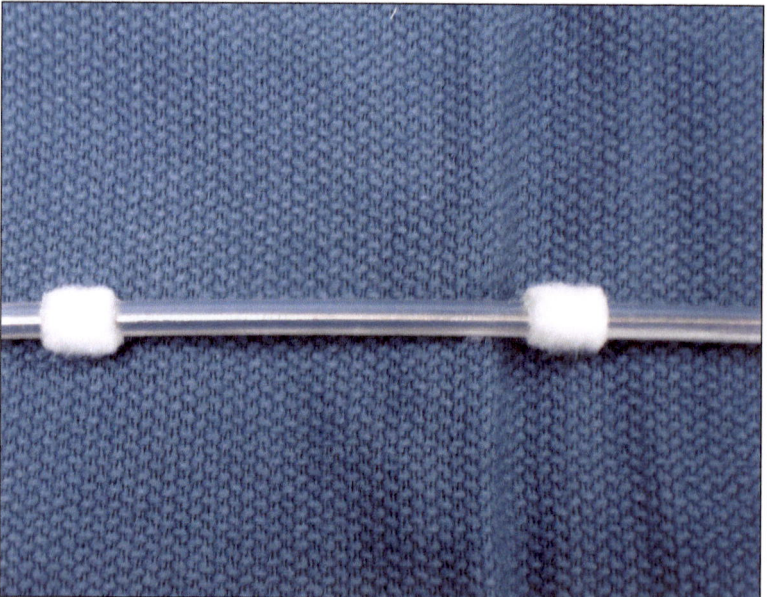

Figure 2.17. The Stylet Sliding into the Catheter Past the Two Dacron cuffs.

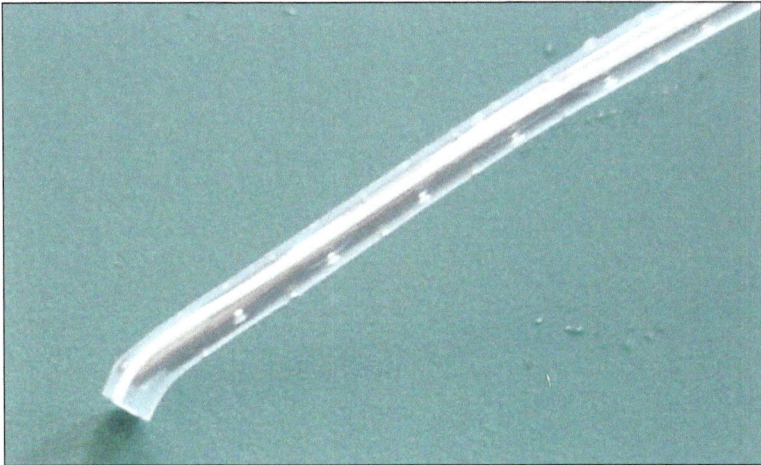

Figure 2.18. The Distal End of the Catheter with the Stylet Properly Inserted
This is the ideal position of the stylet as it is inserted through the small peritoneal incision. Stopping the stylet just short of the end of the catheter minimizes the risk of injuries to visceral structures.

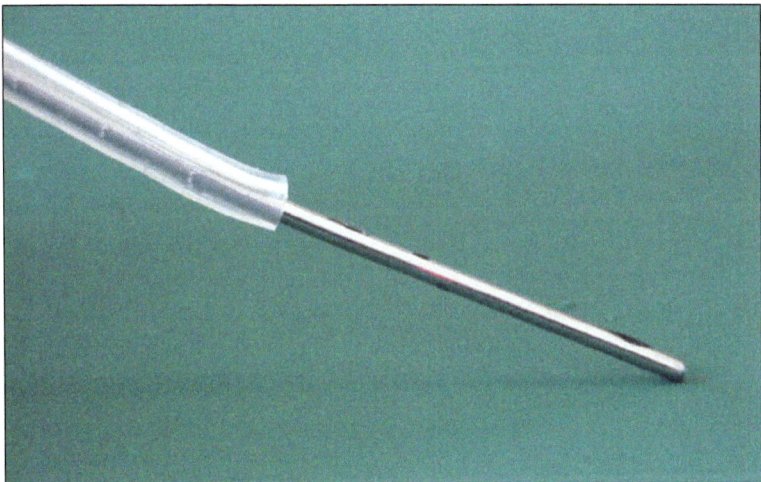

Figure 2.19. Improper (Protruding) Insertion of the Stiffening Stylet
Inserting the catheter with the stylet protruding is dangerous and lends itself to intraperitoneal visceral injuries.

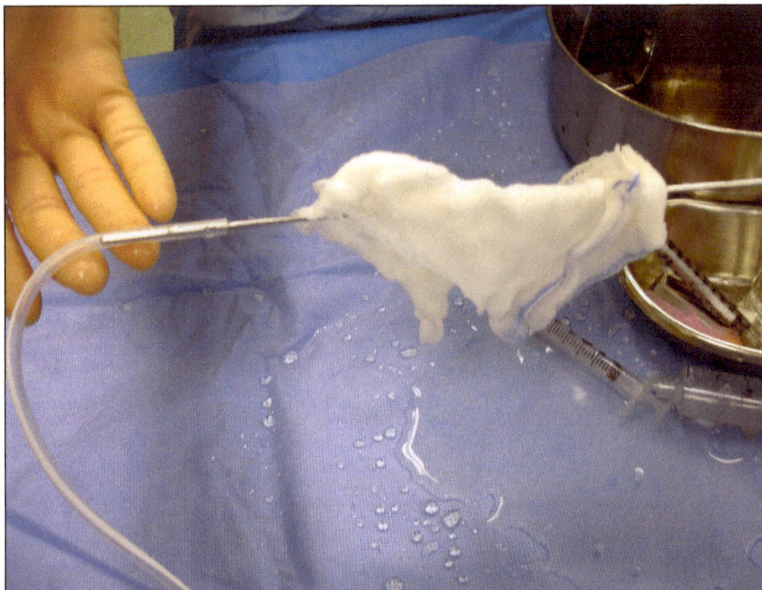

Figure 2.20. Stiffening Stylet Dampened with Wet Gauze
The insertion and later removal of the stiff stylet is facilitated by dripping wet gauze, which keeps the stylet wet ("greased") as it goes into the PD tube. Insertion and removal of the stylet in a dry situation is almost impossible and can result in unpredicted movements with potential injuries. Surgical lubrication gel applied to the stiffening stylet greatly facilitates stylet insertion and removal.

10. Insert the stylet-stiffened catheter through the peritoneal opening. Let the catheter slide down along the anterior abdominal wall. Force must not be used. If resistance is encountered, back up and adjust the direction. When the straightened catheter is 5–10 cm inside the abdomen, retract the stylet 5–10 cm to allow the distal coiled portion of the catheter to resume its coiled state. This insures that the sharp end of the stiff stylet has not slipped beyond the end of the catheter, and leaves the stylet in a position to safely lodge the catheter into the pelvic area. Should resistance occur, redirection of the catheter is attempted until the pelvic area is reached.

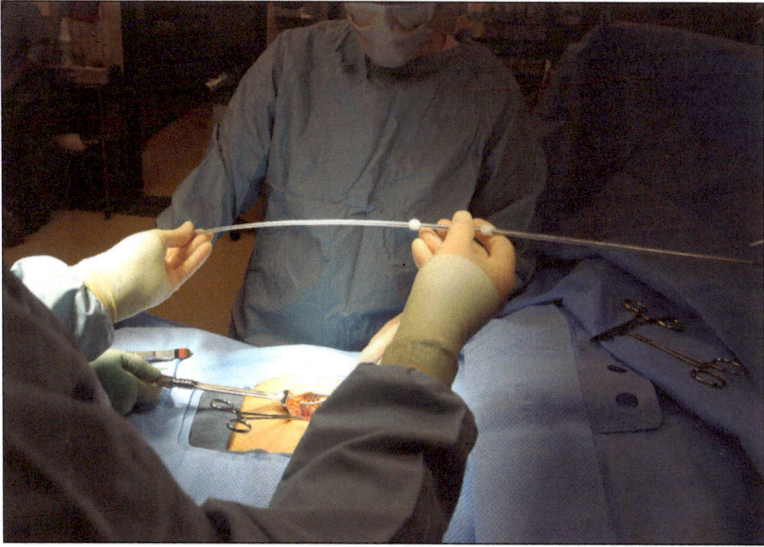

Figure 2.21. Two Cuff, Coiled Catheter with Stiffening Stylet Fully Inserted

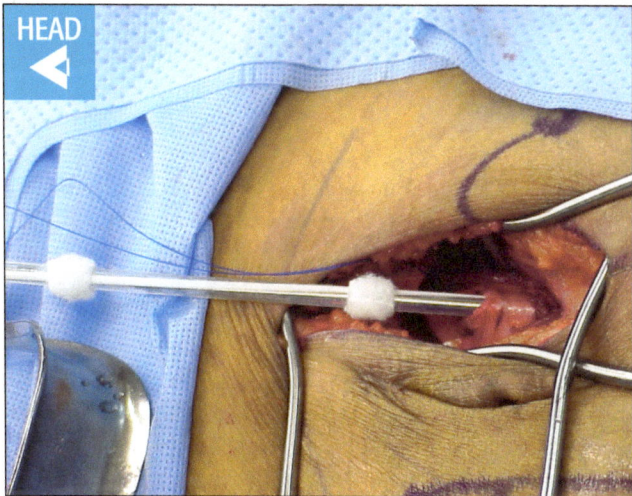

Figure 2.22. Catheter Insertion
The catheter insertion is in progress. At this point, the stiff
stylet has been pulled back a few cm allowing the intra-
abdominal segment of the catheter to become coiled,
facilitating the safe pelvic positioning.

■ 11. When the coiled intra-abdominal segment is in the pelvis, and with 1 hand holding the PD catheter in place at the exit site, pull the stylet out. Tie a purse-string suture snugly around the catheter (Figure 2.23). One should be able to slide the catheter (with some resistance) into position with the Dacron cuff resting onto the posterior rectus fascia.

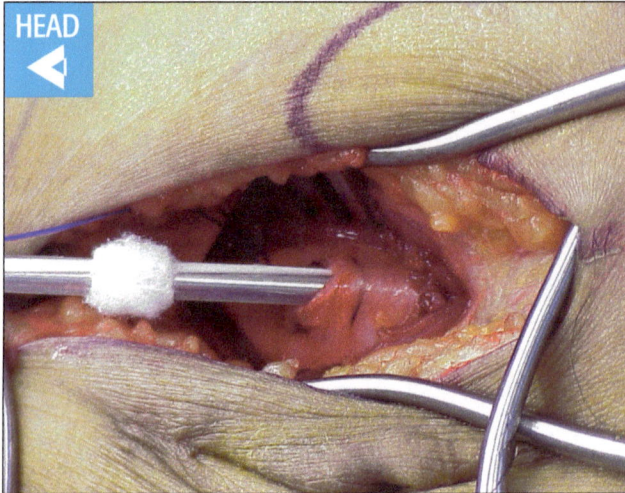

Figure 2.23. Purse-string Suture (Prolene Suture) Tied around the Catheter (Step 11)

■ 12. Using the same purse-string suture, anchor the Dacron cuff with a stitch, entering at the bottom of the cuff and exiting in the posterior aspect (back side) of the cuff. Care must be taken not to puncture the silastic tubing which would cause a permanent leak at the site. The peritoneal cuff will be pushed down to rest on the posterior rectus muscle fascia allowing the stitch through the cuff to be tied (Figure 2.24). Because the catheter maintains its shape and resists sharp bends, and because the peritoneal cuff is aligned parallel to the anterior abdominal wall, the coiled intra-abdominal segment maintains its pelvic position.

■ 13. Using the 20 ml syringe, inject 20–60 ml of saline into the catheter. Test for obstructions to flow by aspirating gently or just draining by gravity. Adjust the catheter placement until good drainage function is achieved.

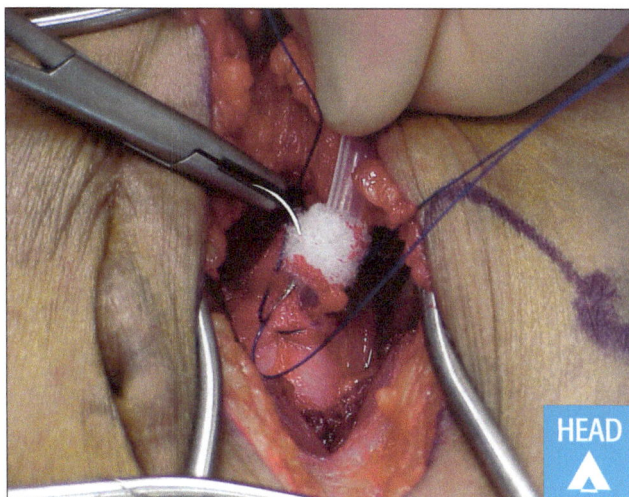

Figure 2.24. The Purse-string Suture, Tied but Not Cut (Step 12)
The Prolene suture is now stitched through the posterior aspect of the Dacron cuff, care taken not to penetrate the catheter itself. The stitch is placed parallel with the tubing in the outward direction.

14. With the 10 ml syringe, inject 0.25% Marcaine (without epinephrine) to anesthetize the rectus muscle, fascia structures, and the subcutaneous tissue and tract. Insert the needle into tissue inside of the wound to avoid contamination from skin bacteria. The Marcaine will also provide postoperative pain control for 8 to 12 hours. By administering the anesthesia now, the risk of inadvertently sticking the catheter is eliminated.

15. Using a Richardson (or US Army) retractor, retract the skin and subcutaneous tissue upwards exposing the anterior rectus fascia. Using a mosquito or a right angle hemostat, penetrate (from the outside) the anterior fascia 2–3 cm directly above the upper edge of the anterior rectus fascia incision. Vertical alignment of the hemostat penetration and the hole in the peritoneum is critical to maintaining proper vertical alignment of the intra-abdominal segment. Clamp onto the end of the catheter and pull it behind and through the rectus muscle and the anterior fascia (Figures 2.25 and 2.26). Using a hemostat, the anterior rectus fascia is widened somewhat to allow passage of the subcutaneous Dacron cuff that will be placed just under the skin near the skin exit site (Figure 2.27).

Once the cuff is pulled to its final position through the fascia for placement 1.5–2.0 cm inside of the skin exit site (Figures 2.28 and 2.29), the direction of the peritoneal cuff and catheter will be aligned parallel to the anterior abdominal wall, which will place and keep the coiled portion of the catheter in the pelvic area. At this point, the PD catheter is aligned straight behind the rectus muscle.

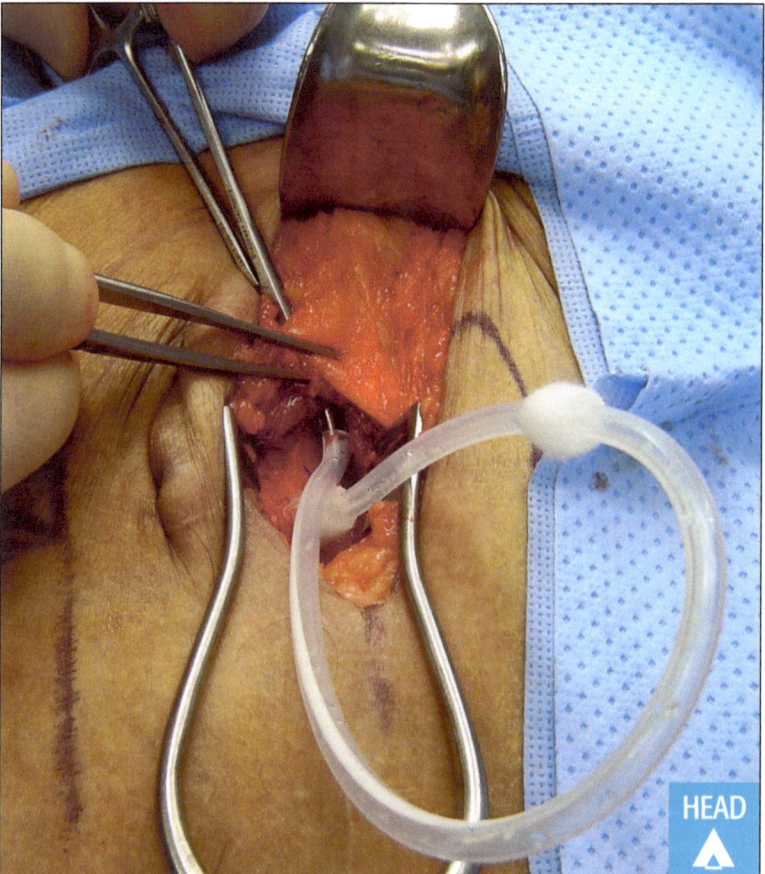

Figure 2.25. Mosquito Hemostat Penetrating the Fascia and Pulling the Catheter Through

A mosquito hemostat is used to penetrate the anterior rectus fascia about 2–3 cm above the upper corner of the external rectus fascia incision. The catheter is grabbed and pulled through the anterior rectus muscle fascia.

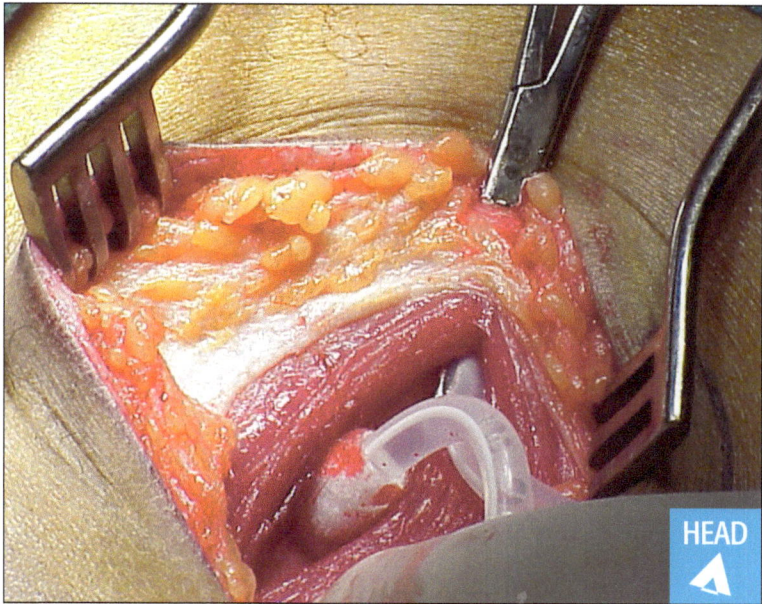

Figure 2.26. Hemostat Pulling the Catheter through the Fascia (Step 15)
This close up image details the catheter's direction and relationship to the abdominal anatomic structures as it is pulled with a hemostat through the fascia. Vertical alignment (parallel to the body) of the site where the catheter exits the peritoneum and the hole through the external rectus fascia penetrated by the hemostat is critical in maintaining the vertical alignment of the catheter and the proper location for the coiled portion in the pelvis.

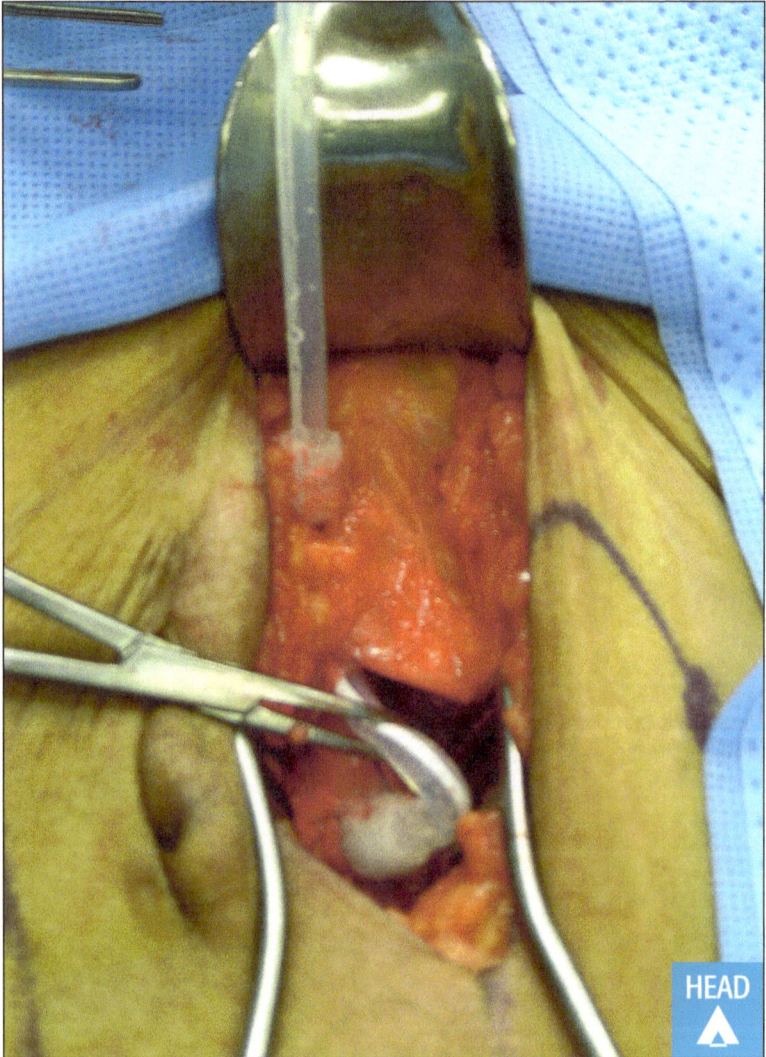

Figure 2.27. External Dacron Cuff as it Exits the Fascia (Step 15)
This image shows both Dacron cuffs, the subcutaneous just being pulled through the anterior rectus muscle fascia. The peritoneal cuff and catheter is temporarily out of vertical alignment while being pulled through the anterior rectus muscle fascia.

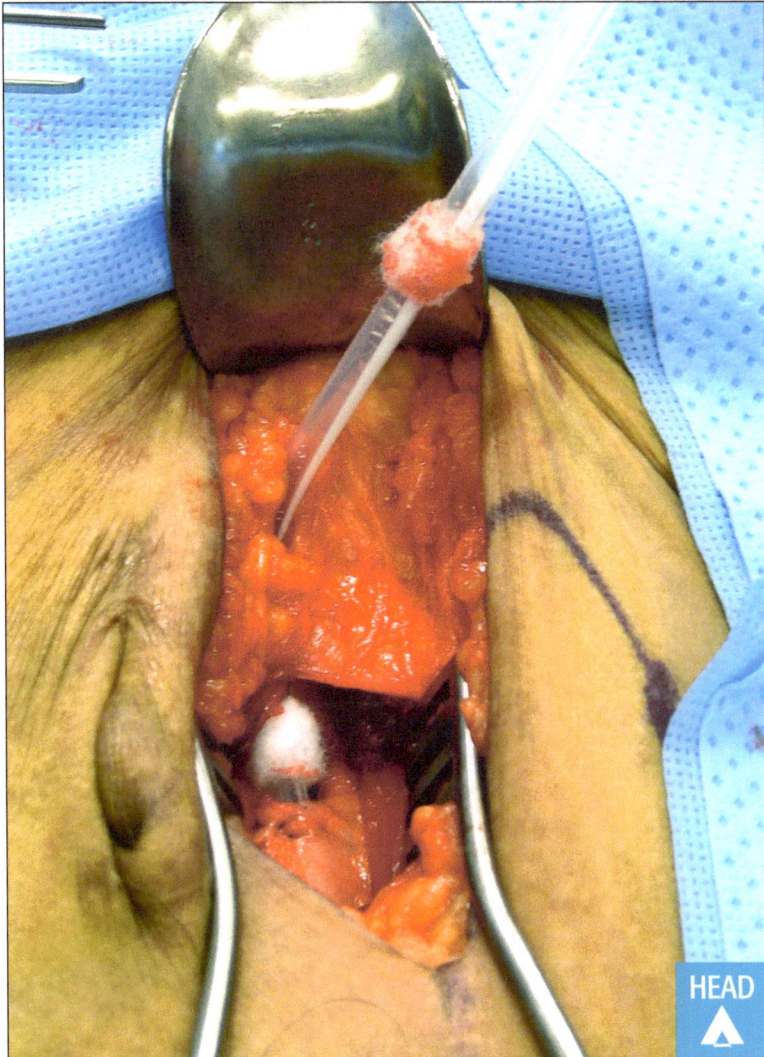

Figure 2.28. Catheter Ready for Tunneling to Exit Site (Step 16)
The peritoneal Dacron cuff now rests on and is sutured to the posterior rectus muscle fascia. The catheter is aligned in a cephalad direction keeping the coiled portion in a downward direction, toward the pelvis and away from omentum structures. Downward bowel peristalsis on the left side will also facilitate maintaining the pelvic position of the catheter.

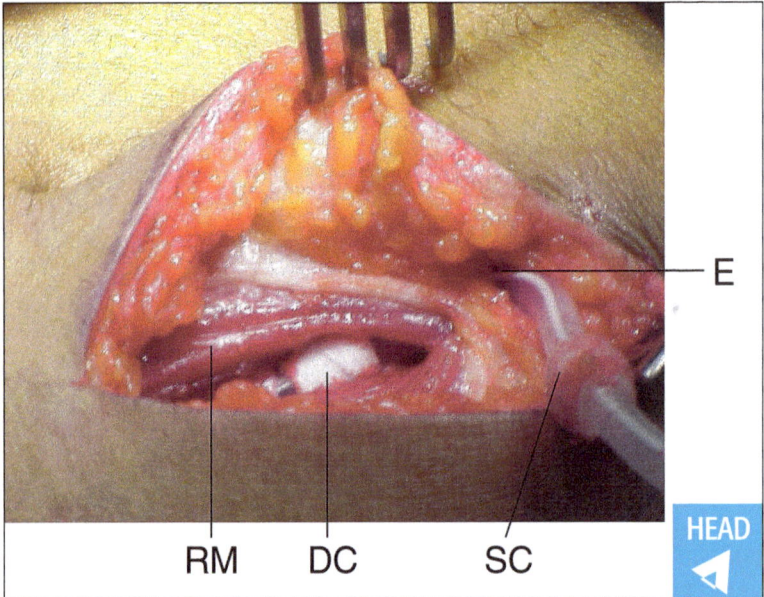

Figure 2.29. Close up of Catheter Ready for Tunneling to Exit Site
The catheter has been pulled from the pre-peritoneum and posterior rectus fascia through the rectus muscle and the anterior rectus sheath. The peritoneal Dacron cuff (DC) sits outside the posterior rectus fascia behind the rectus muscle (RM). The catheter is inserted through the anterior rectus fascia at E, and ready to be tunneled through the skin at the predetermined site. The subcutaneous Dacron cuff (SC) will be located 1.5–2 cm, from the skin exit site. These next critical steps are detailed in Figures 2.31–2.32.

Because of their very sharp needle-like edge, tunnelers (Figure 2.30) must be protected with a plastic cover when not in use. Great care must be taken to avoid injuring operating room personnel. The surgeon should handle the subcutaneous tunneling steps with no help or interference from other team members.

16. Attach the subcutaneous tunneler (Figure 2.30) to the catheter (Figure 2.31). By properly directing the tunneler, a smooth lumen will be formed as it tunnels subcutaneously along the marked path and exits through the skin. Insert the sharp tip under the edge of the incision and work the tunneler along the marked path through the subcutaneous tissue and out the exit site. Pull the tubing through the exit site until the subcutaneous Dacron cuff rests 1.5–2.0 cm inside the exit site. A snug fit between catheter and skin at the exit site will hold the cuff in place making migration through the skin unlikely.

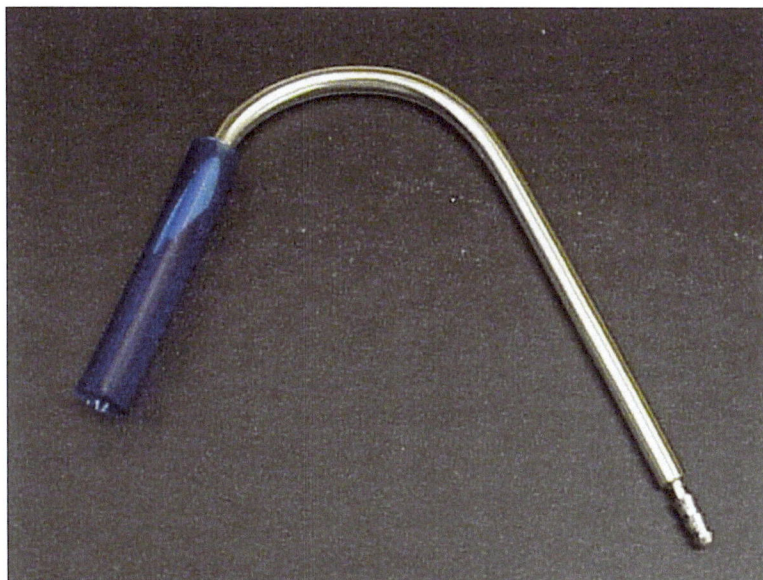

Figure 2.30. The Blake 15FR Drain Trocar
The Blake 15FR drain trocar (with the plastic drain removed) is an alternative to the Faller tunneler. The barbed edges at the end (lower right corner) fit snugly into the plastic Tenckhoff catheter and can be pulled through the subcutaneous tissues without the tube becoming dislodged (Step 16). The Faller tunneler requires a tie around the PD catheter that may still slip off requiring repeated, unnecessary trauma to the exit site.

The tunneler should exit the skin at an angle of about 30 to 45 degrees in order to optimize catheter-to-skin alignment and comfort for the patient (Figure 2.33).

A tunneler with the same diameter as the catheter tubing prevents migration of the subcutaneous cuff and eliminates the need for stitches to anchor the catheter tube at the exit site. No stitches should be placed at the exit site. Stitches create tension, which causes pain and trauma, promoting infection at the exit site. Also, when stitches have been placed the patients sometimes think they are permanent and fail to return to have them removed.

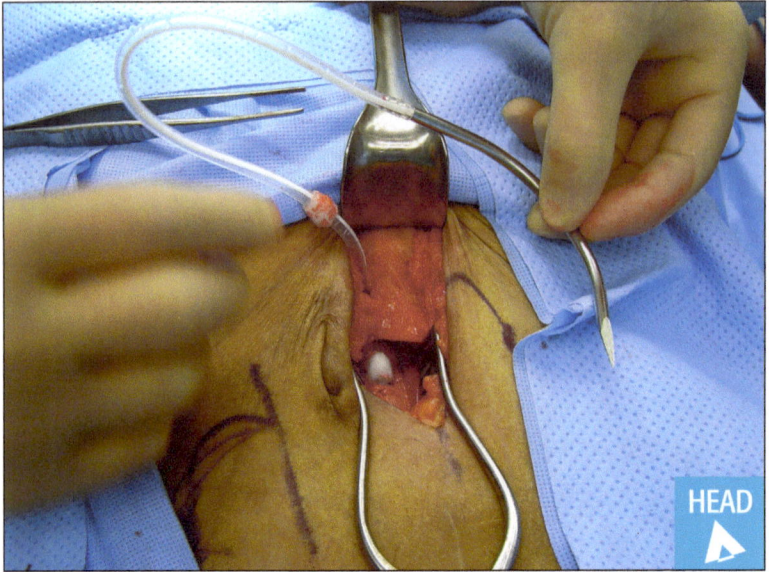

Figure 2.31. Tunneler Attached to the Catheter (Step 16)
The peritoneal cuff is aligned parallel with the anterior abdominal wall. The subcutaneous tunneler is attached to the catheter in preparation for tunneling along the marked exit path and out the exit site.

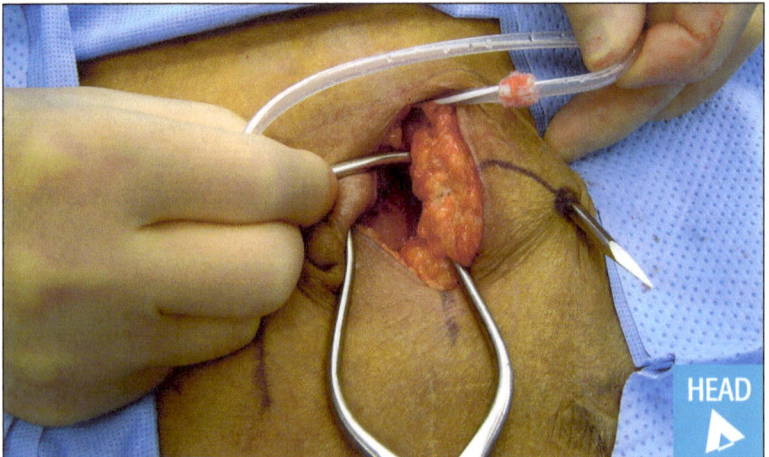

Figure 2.32. Tunneler Emerging from the Marked Exit Site (Step 16)
The tunneler has penetrated the skin at the predetermined and marked site, breaking the skin at an angle of about 30–45 degrees.

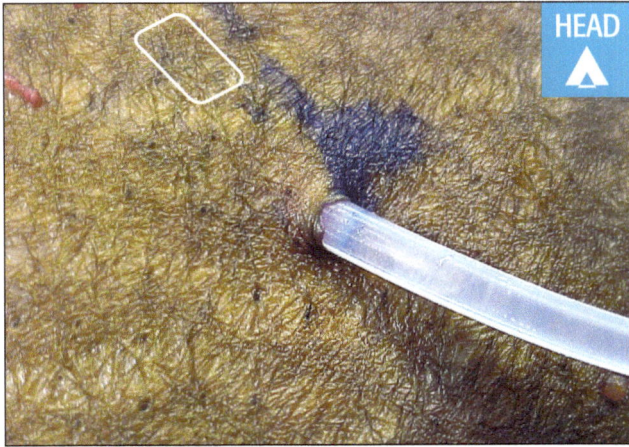

Figure 2.33. Detail of the Skin Exit Site
This close up image of the catheter exit site shows a snug fit with no bleeding, no stitches, and minimal trauma—thereby minimizing risk for postoperative infectious complications. The subcutaneous cuff is indicated by the white outline. The key to a snug fit is in choosing a tunneling device that is of the same or similar diameter as the catheter tube. It cannot be stressed enough, that stitches must NOT be placed at the exit site to "anchor" the catheter.

An alternative to puncturing the exit site with the tunneler from the inside is to use a skin biopsy punch (Figure 2.34). A 3 mm punch appears to be the ideal size as it creates a tight exit that fits snugly around the catheter (Figures 2.33–2.40).

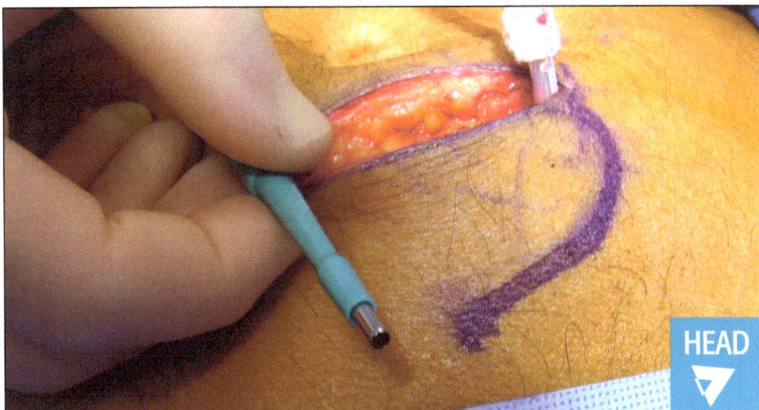

Figure 2.34. Skin Biopsy Punch, 3 mm

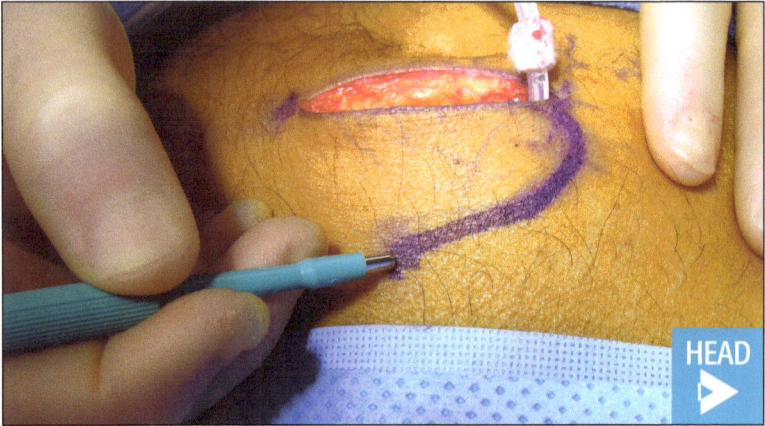

Figure 2.35. Skin Biopsy Punch Penetrating the Skin
Rotate the punch to gently cut through the skin at an angle of about 45 degrees.

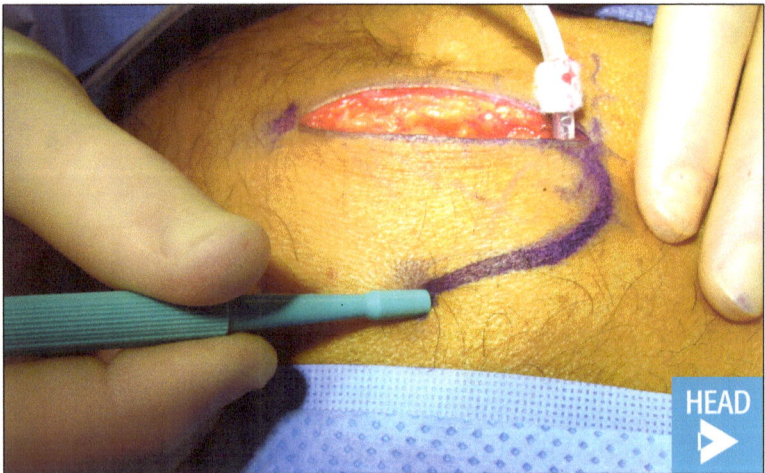

Figure 2.36. Skin Biopsy Punch Fully Penetrating the Skin
It is not necessary to reach the base of the puncher as shown in this image, as it may induce unnecessary bleeding.

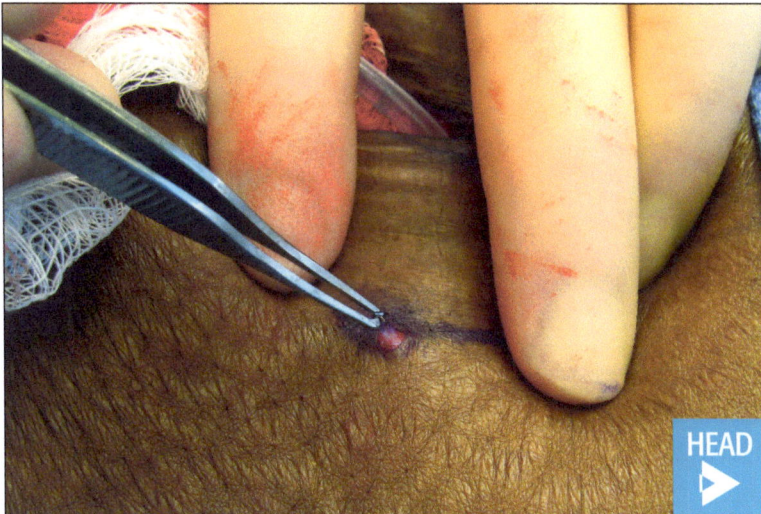

Figure 2.37. Punched Skin Tag Held by Forceps for Removal
The punched skin tag remains attached at its base and must be removed. Clasp with forceps and carefully cut it off.

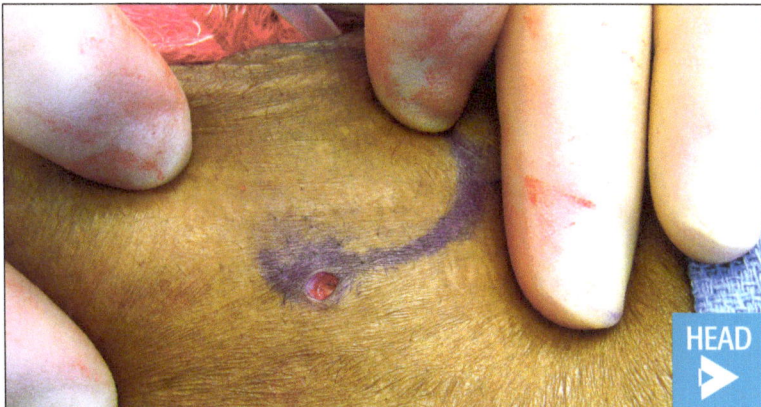

Figure 2.38. Completed Skin Biopsy Punch
The skin biopsy punch creates a small skin exit lumen that fits snugly around the PD catheter.

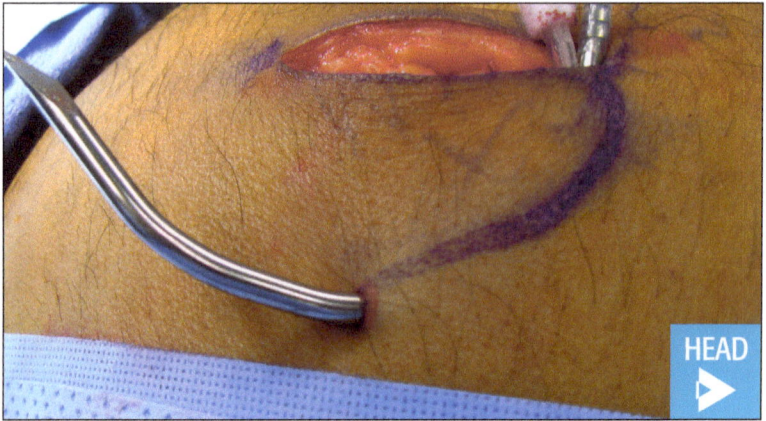

Figure 2.39. Tunneler Exiting Through a Lumen Made with a Skin Biopsy Punch
Close up image of the subcutaneous tunneler as it exits the hole made by the 3 mm skin biopsy punch. The punch is the same diameter as the PD catheter. The skin punch tends to eliminate the bleeding that sometimes occurs when the sharp edges of the tunneler cut through the skin exit site.

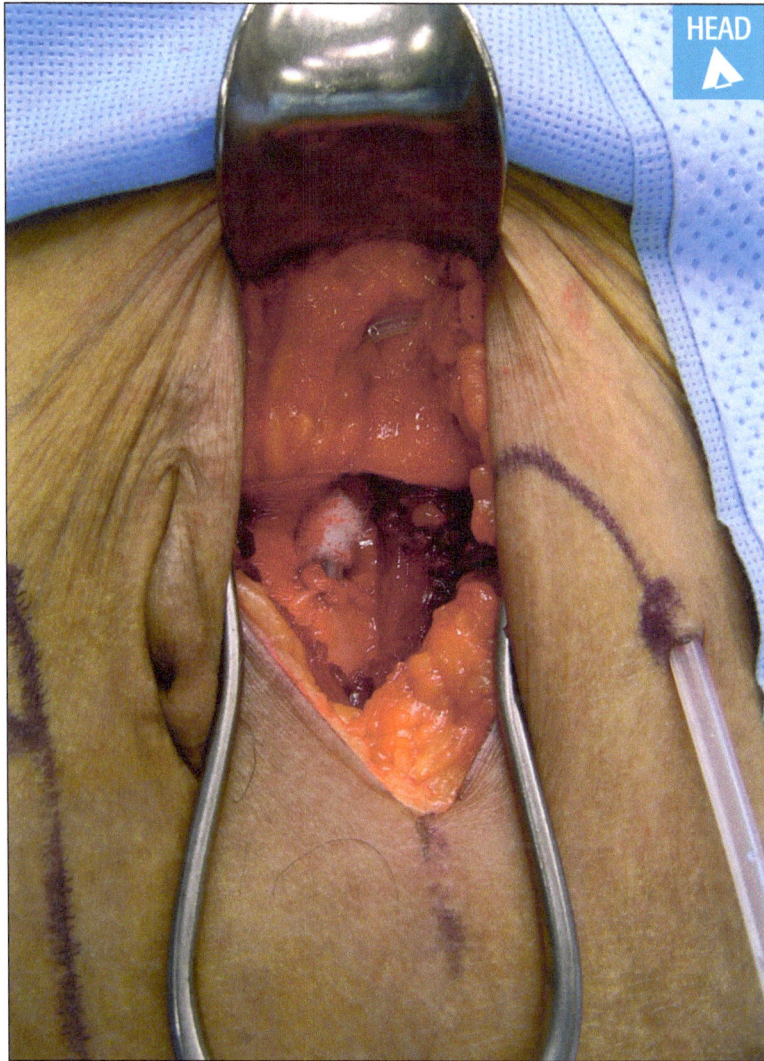

Figure 2.40. The Catheter in Place

This image illustrates important technical aspects of the surgical anatomy. The peritoneal cuff is attached to the posterior fascia with the catheter aligned vertically as it ascends through the anterior rectus fascia, thereby keeping the coiled portion in the pelvic area. A smooth subcutaneous arched path between the Dacron cuffs. A snug catheter exit site, with the subcutaneous Dacron cuff (not visible) 1.5–2.0 cm inside the skin exit site.

Under no circumstances should a knife incision be made to force a hemostat retrograde to catch and pull the catheter out through the skin. This technique induces bleeding and can be quite traumatic to the skin, requiring stitches. The trauma and stitches can cause complications and infection at the exit site (Figure 2.41).

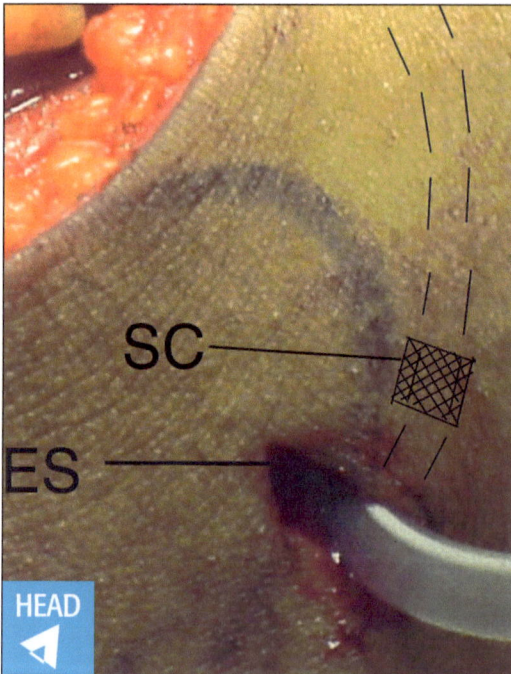

Figure 2.41. Example of an Incorrectly Executed Exit Site
This image illustrates incorrect technique. The catheter exit site (ES) incision is too large and will require a stitch to stop the bleeding and to prevent the subcutaneous cuff (SC) from migrating.

17. Using the 20 ml syringe (Figure 2.42), inject 20–60 ml of saline into the catheter to make sure there are no kinks or obstructions to flow. Test the flow by aspirating gently or just drain by gravity. Rapid, unobstructed drainage function must be achieved. Leave 40–60 ml of saline in the abdomen in preparation for the next step.

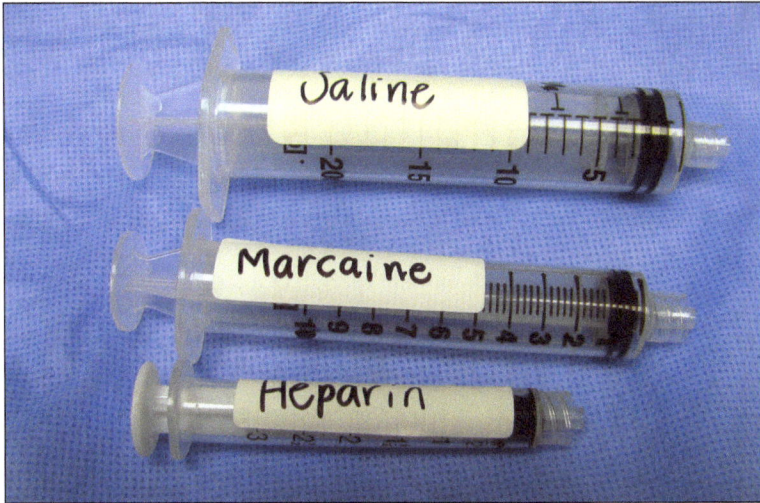

Figure 2.42. Syringes Labeled for Safety and Convenience
During PD catheter placement, 3 syringes are used for very different purposes. The 20 ml syringe is filled with saline and used to flush large volumes through the catheter. The 10 ml syringe is used for injecting local anesthesia: 0.25% Marcaine. The 5 ml syringe is used to inject a small volume (3.5 ml Heparin 1000 units/ml) to prime the PD catheter and the coiled portion exit holes. The consistent use of syringes in 3 different sizes removes confusion, increases safety, and makes the volume infused match the size of the syringe. (For example, it is difficult, unsafe, and inaccurate to inject 3.5 ml of heparin, 1000 Units /ml, with a 20 ml or 10 ml syringe.)

18. Gather the 3 occlusion pieces that come in the catheter kit: a luer end piece, a cap for the luer piece, and a clamp (Figure 2.43). Insert the ridged or barbed end of the luer piece into the end of the catheter tube with rotating movements while applying pressure on the luer piece. Insert the 5 ml syringe containing heparin into the luer piece and inject 3.5–4.0 ml of heparin (concentration 1000 units/ml) to prevent catheter obstruction from small blood clots or fibrin. The heparin now fills the 3.2 ml lumen volume of the 62.5 cm 2-cuff catheter, including the coiled portion. Leave the heparin syringe attached and clamp the tube midway with the catheter occlusion clamp to suspend the heparin in the catheter and prevent the heparin from leaking out the luer end or from flowing into the abdomen and defeating the purpose. The 40–60 ml of saline retained in the abdominal cavity in step 17 helps to suspend the heparin in the targeted areas. Remove the 5 ml syringe and twist the cap onto the luer insert.

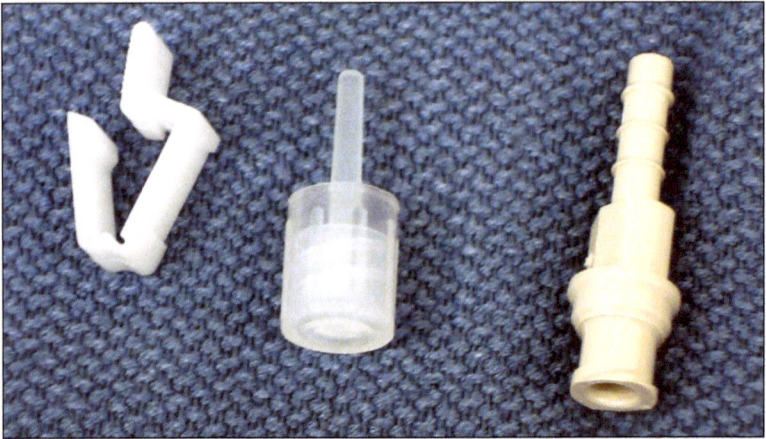

Figure 2.43. Catheter Kit Occlusion Pieces (Step 18)
From left to right: a clamp for closing flow, a cap with plug that screws onto the luer end piece, a luer end piece that is inserted into the catheter tube. Open the catheter kit with care, as these small pieces are easily lost.

Closing the Wound

19. Close the anterior rectus muscle fascia with a size 2-0 Prolene Suture on a SH needle (Figure 2.44), applied in a running fashion, with tightly spaced stitches for a "watertight" seal (Figure 2.45).

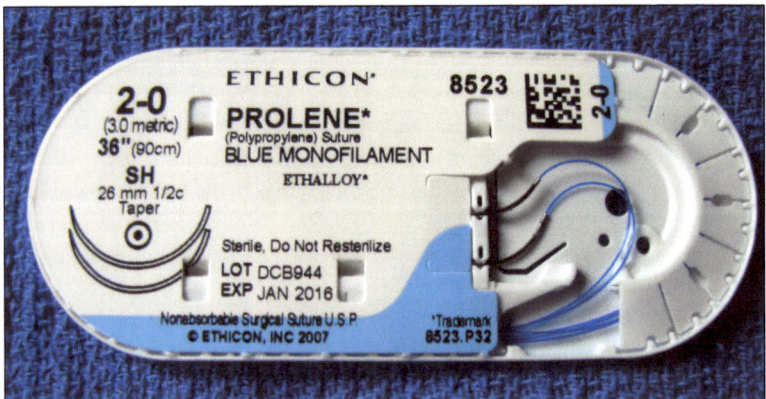

Figure 2.44. Non-absorbable Suture with Needle (Prolene Suture, 2-0, SH needle)
The fascia is closed with a non-absorbable suture.

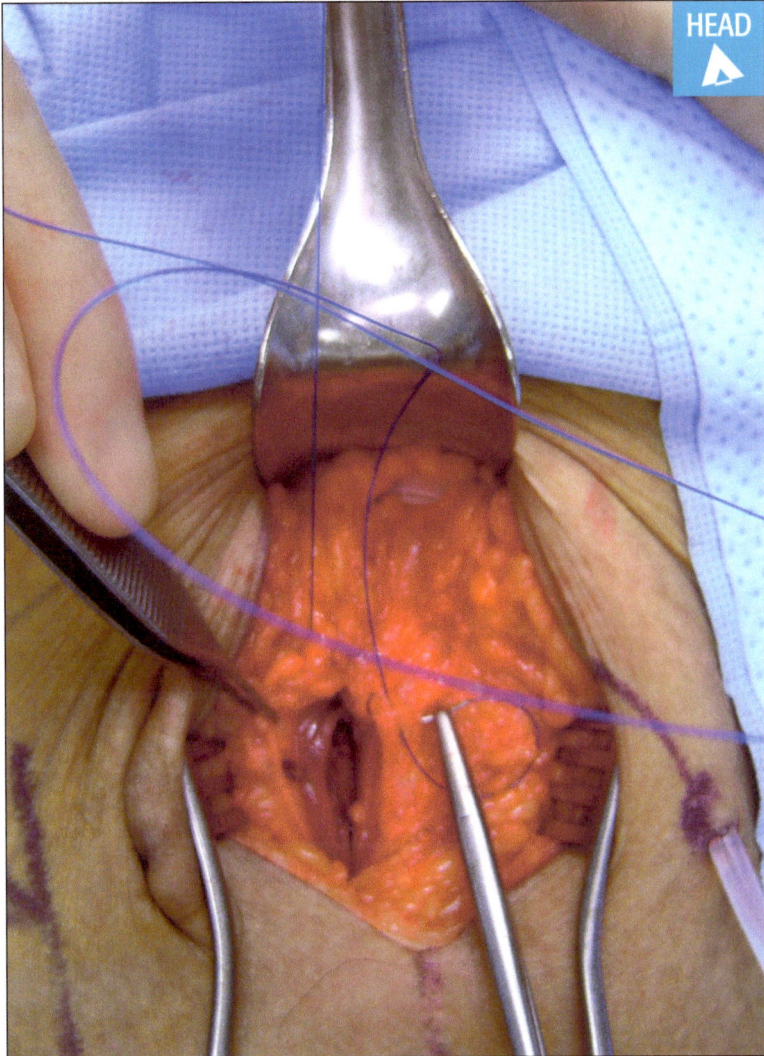

Figure 2.45. Suturing of the Anterior Rectus Fascia (Step 19)
After obtaining exact hemostasis, the anterior rectus muscle fascia is closed with a running suture (Prolene Suture, 2-0, SH needle).

■ 20. Suture the skin incision using a size 4-0 or 5-0 absorbable suture with a 1/2 circle, taper point, 17 mm needle (PDS Suture, size 4-0 or 5-0, RB-1 needle; Ethicon, USA) (Figure 2.46)—making 3–4 interrupted, inverted sutures to align the skin edges without strangulation. In most instances, no deep subcutaneous sutures are needed (Figure 2.47). Make sure that the last knot is positioned so that the suture ends will not stick through the skin.

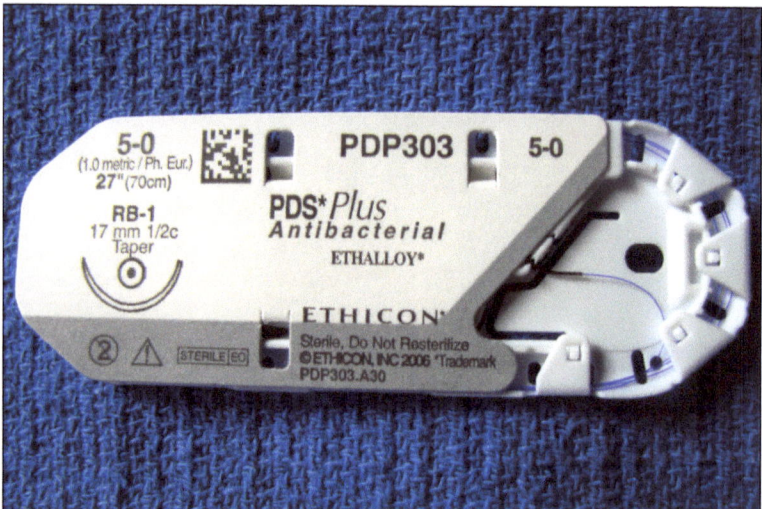

Figure 2.46. Absorbable Suture with Needle (PDS Suture, 5-0, RB-1 needle)
The skin is closed with 5-0 PDS Suture on a RB-1 needle. The RB-1 is a non-cutting needle, which causes less bleeding as it penetrates tissues and skin.

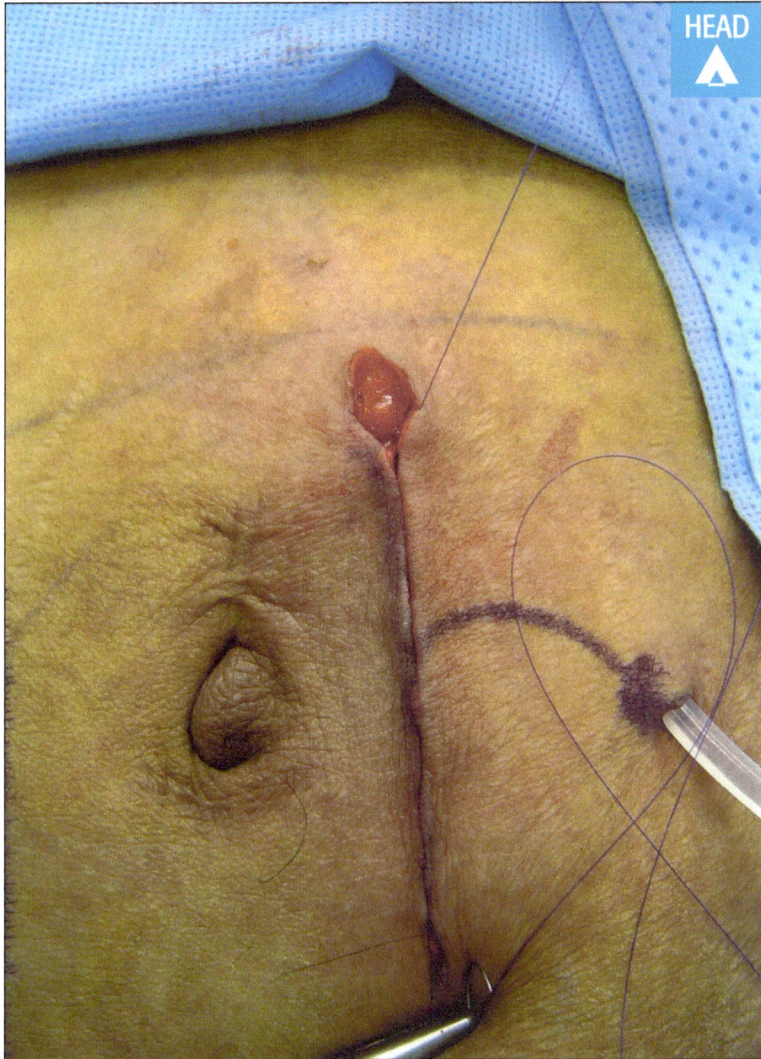

Figure 2.47. Subcuticular Suture Closing the Skin Incision
A subcuticular suture closing the skin may not improve cosmetics when compared with 3–4 inverted properly placed sutures. Minimal tension on the sutures prevents skin ischemia and promotes healing.

■ 21. Dressing the PD catheter wound involves several important steps. Suggested dressing material is pictured in Figure 2.48. Benzoin or a liquid adhesive (Mastisol Liquid Adhesive; Ferndale Pharma Group, Ferndale, MI) helps to adhere a longitudinal, adhesive sterile closure strip on the incision (Steri-Strip; Nexcare Products/3M, USA) (Figure 2.49). Place a folded, incised gauze around the catheter at the exit site (Figure 2.50). Place a second folded piece of gauze on top of the Steri-Strip (Figure 2.50). An extra layer of gauze will prevent the catheter and clamp from coming in contact with the skin (Figure 2.51). One or two adhesive film dressings are placed over the gauze, and the catheter is rolled up on top of the transparent film, making sure no catheter part or clamp is in contact with the skin (Figure 2.52). Place gauze over the rolled up catheter to facilitate removal and dressing changes (Figure 2.53). Place 2–3 adhesive film dressings over the gauze, taking care to avoid adhering the film to the catheter (Figure 2.54). One or two more transparent film dressings may be needed for a complete seal.

The most important aspect of postoperative management is to keep the area dry and free from moisture. Properly placed the patient can take a shower without the dressing getting wet. The dressing may be left in place for 5–7 days. If the dressing becomes soiled, soaked, or begins to peel away, it must be replaced.

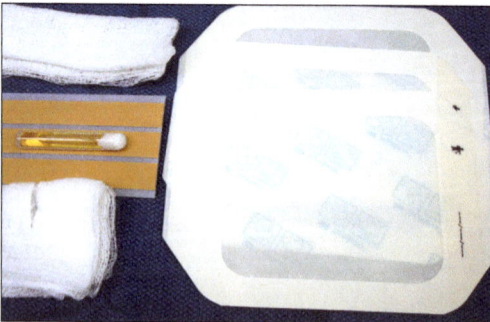

Figure 2.48.   Recommended Dressing Supplies
Several pieces of 4 × 4 gauze, (3) 10 mm × 100 mm Steri-Strips, benzoin or Mastisol Liquid Adhesive, and 3–4 sheets of transparent dressing 10 cm x 12 cm (Tegaderm Waterproof Transparent Dressing; Nexcare Products/3M, USA)

Steri-Strips applied transverse or across the incision tend to cause skin blistering if applied under tension. Also, if transverse strips are removed too early, the skin edges may accidentally be pulled part.

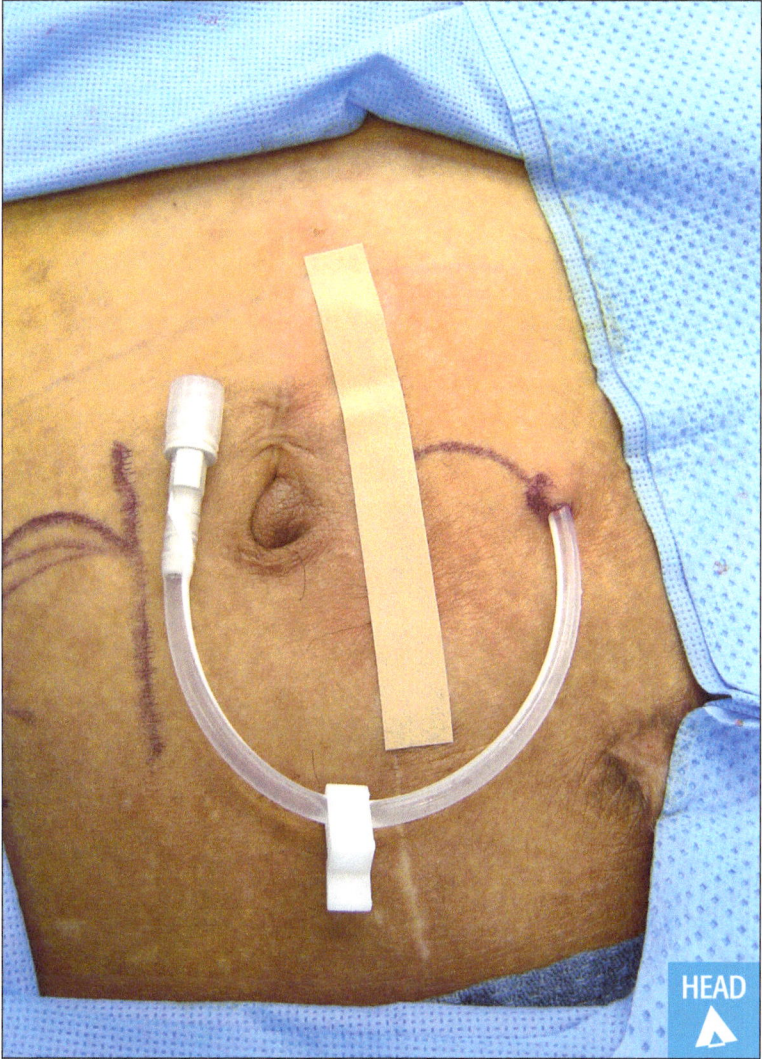

Figure 2.49. Site Ready for Dressing (Step 21)
The catheter with the clamp (occluding the catheter) and cap in place. One longitudinal, sterile adhesive strip covers the incision.

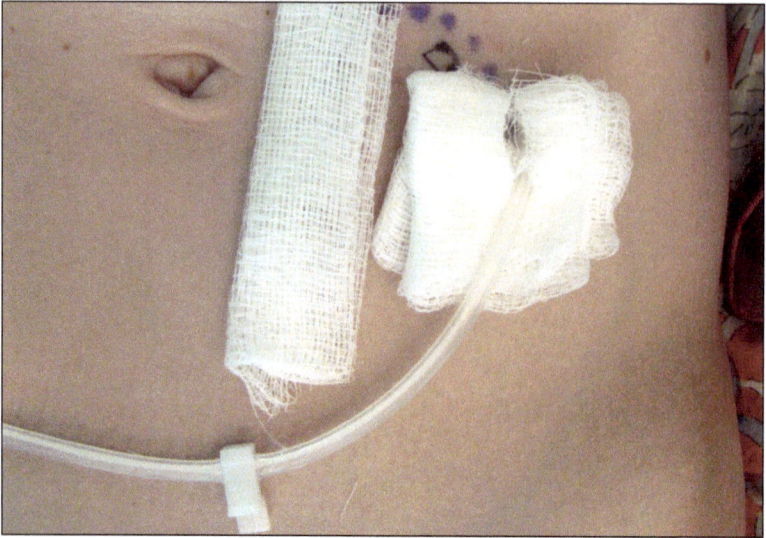

Figure 2.50. First Layer of Gauze in Place
A 2 × 2 inch piece of gauze is cut from one side to the center and placed around the catheter at the exit site to avoid catheter-to-skin direct contact. The incision is covered with a 2 × 4 inch gauze dressing.

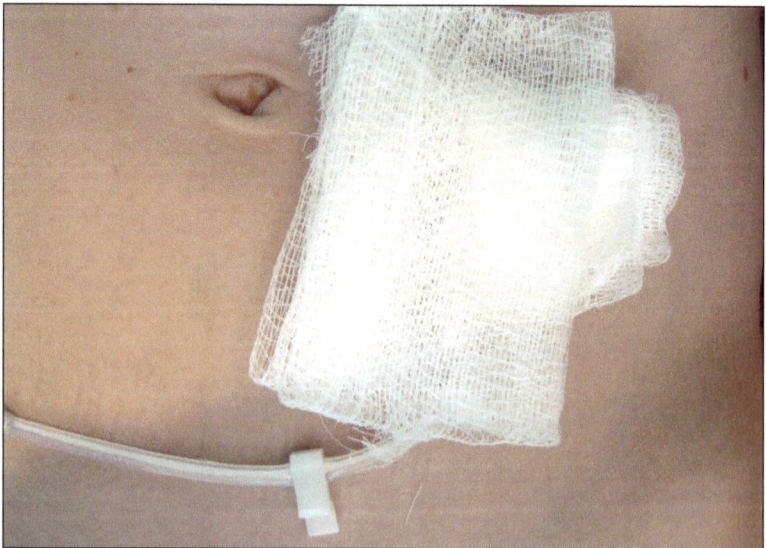

Figure 2.51. Second Layer of Gauze in Place

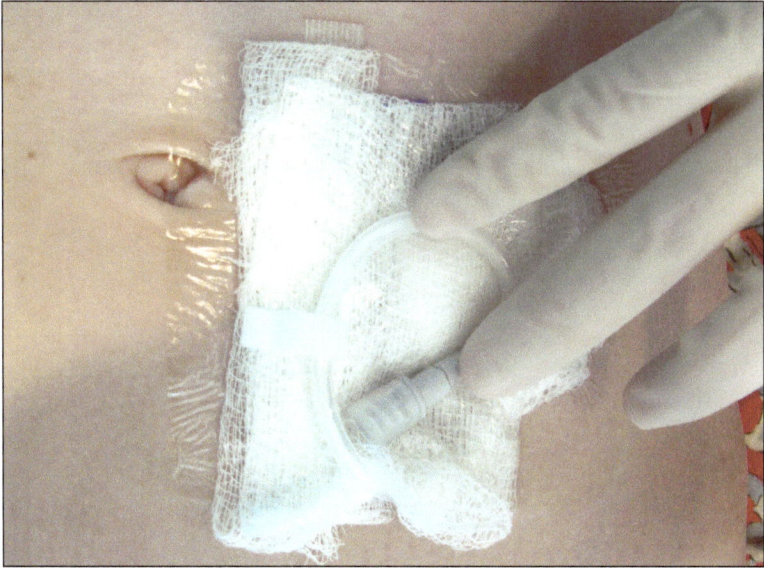

Figure 2.52. First Layer of Adhesive Film Dressing Applied
The external portion of the catheter is rolled up and placed on top of the adhesive film.

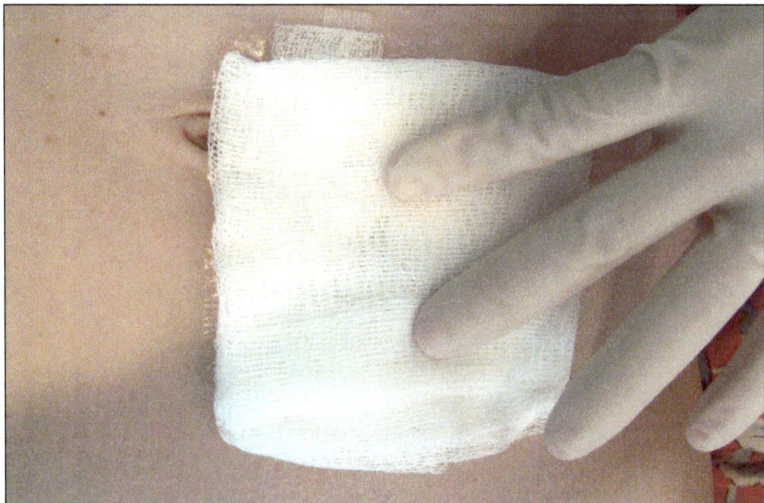

Figure 2.53. Third Layer of Gauze Applied
This gauze layer is to prevent the adhesive dressing from sticking to the catheter. Once adhered, the film is hard to separate from the catheter, making removal of the dressing difficult and even dangerous.

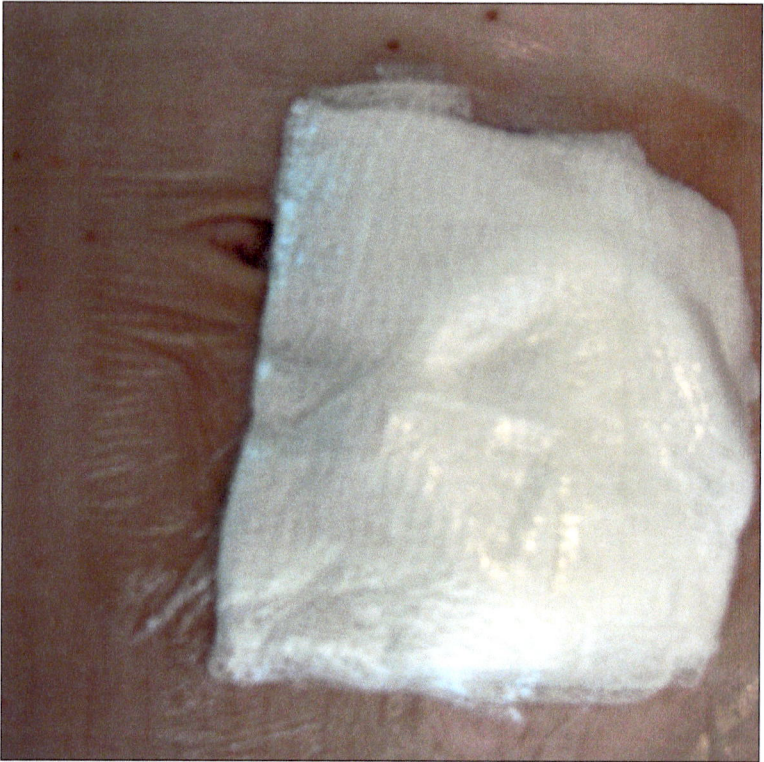

Figure 2.54. Dressing Complete
The area is covered with additional adhesive film dressing for a "watertight" seal, allowing the patient to shower. The catheter itself and the occluding clamp must not be in contact with the skin.

REFERENCES

1.   Eklund B, Honkanen E, Kyllonem L, et al. Peritoneal dialysis access: prospective randomized comparison of single-cuff and double-cuff straight Tenckhoff catheters. *Nephrol Dial Transplant* 1997, 12: 2664.

2.   Gokal R, Alexander S, Ash S, et al. Peritoneal catheters and exit-site practices toward optimum peritoneal access: 1998 update. *Perit Dial Int* 1998, 18: 11.

3.   Flanigan M, Gokal R. Peritoneal catheters and exit-site practices toward optimum peritoneal access: a review of current developments. *Perit Dial Int* 2005, 25: 132.

4.   Nessim SJ, Bargman JM, Jassal SV. Relationship between double-cuff versus single-cuff peritoneal dialysis catheters and risk of peritonitis. *Nephrol Dial Transplant* 2010, 25: 2310.

5.   Di Paolo N, Capotondo L, Sansoni E, et al. The self-locating catheter: clinical experience and follow-up. *Perit Dial Int* 2004, 24:359.

6.   Singh N, Davidson I, Minhajuddin A, et al. Risk factors associated with peritoneal dialysis catheter survival: a 9-year single-center study in 315 patients. *J Vasc Access* 2010, 11: 316.

7.   Crabtree JH, Burchette RJ. Effect of prior abdominal surgery, peritonitis, and adhesions on catheter function and long-term outcomes on peritoneal dialysis. *Am Surg* 2009, 75: 140.

8.   Gadallah MF, Pervez A, El-Shahawy MA, et al. Peritoneoscopic versus surgical placement of peritoneal dialysis catheters: a prospective randomized study of outcome. *Am J Kidney Dis* 1999, 33: 118.

9.   Jwo SC, Chen KS, Lee CC, et al. Prospective randomized study for comparison of open surgery with laparoscopic-assisted placement of Tenckhoff peritoneal dialysis catheter – a single center experience and literature review. *J Surg Res* 2010, 159: 489.

10. Santarelli S, Zeiler M, Marinelli R, et al. Videolaparoscopy as rescue therapy and placement of peritoneal dialysis catheters: a thirty-two case single centre experience. *Nephrol Dial Transplant* 2006, 21: 1348.

11. Crabtree JH, Fishman A. Selective performance of prophylactic omentopexy during laparoscopic implantation of peritoneal dialysis catheters. *Surg Laparoscop Endoscop Percutan Tech* 2003, 13: 180.

12. Dalgic A, Ersoy E, Anderson ME, et al. A novel minimally invasive technique for insertion of peritoneal dialysis catheter. *Surg Laparoscop Endoscop Percutan Tech* 2002, 12: 252.

13. Tsimoyiannis ECT, Siakas P, Glantzounis G, et al. Laparoscopic placement of the Tenckhoff catheter for peritoneal dialysis. *Surg Laparoscop Endosc Percutan Tech* 2000, 10: 218.

14. Wright MJ, Bel'eed K, Johnson BF, et al. Randomized prospective comparison of laparoscopic and open peritoneal dialysis catheter insertion. *Perit Dial Int* 1999, 19: 372.

15. Watson DI, Paterson D, Bannister K. Secure placement of peritoneal dialysis catheters using a laparoscopic technique. *Surg Laparosc Endosc* 1996, 6: 35.

16. Attaluri V, Lebeis C, Brethauer S, et al. Advanced laparoscopic techniques significantly improve function of peritoneal dialysis catheters. *J Am Coll Surg* 2010, 211: 699.

17. Maio R, FIgueiredo N, Costa P. Laparoscopic placement of Tenckhoff catheters for peritoneal dialysis: a safe, effective, and reproducible procedure. *Perit Dial Int* 2008, 28: 170.

18. Zadrozny D, Draczkowski T, Lichodziejewska-Niemierko K. Two-millimeter minisite mini-laparoscopy for rescue of dysfunctional continuous ambulatory peritoneal dialysis catheters. *Surg Laparosc Endosc Percutan* 1999, Tech 9: 369.

SUMMARIZED STEPS FOR OPEN SURGICAL PLACEMENT OF A TWO CUFF, COILED CATHETER

SURGICAL SAFETY AND INSTRUMENTS CHECKLISTS

I. DAVIDSON, K. FRAZIER

This summary of steps is provided as a quick reference for operating room personnel and surgeons to plan and anticipate issues before each surgery. Instruments, supplies, and tools are printed in **red**. For a more detailed operative description of the open peritoneal catheter placement, please see Chapter 2.

Table 3.1. List of Instruments, Supplies, and Drugs

Number in Set	Basic Instrumentation
1	sterile marking pen
1	straight suture scissors
1	regular Metzenbaum scissors
1	fine Metzenbaum scissors
1	Allis forceps
1	tonsil hemostat
2	hemostat - curved
4	Mosquito hemostat - curved
2	Adson forceps - with teeth
2	DeBakey forceps
1	tissue forceps
1	Richardson retractor – baby or medium
1	Weitlaner retractor
1	Weitlaner retractor - baby
2	Senn retractors
1	US Army retractor
2	needle holder - regular
1	#3 knife handle
1	tunneling trocar (Blake Drain 15FR with Trocar – drain removed)
1	skin biopsy punch (optional)
1	stiff stylet for straightening the catheter
1	Tenckhoff catheter - 24 inch, 62.5 cm, 2 cuff

continued on page 60

continued from page 59

1	size 2-0 non-absorbable suture with ½ circle, taper point, 26 mm needle (Prolene 2-0, SH needle)
1	size 5-0 absorbable suture with a ½ circle, taper point, 17 mm needle (PDS Suture 5-0; RB-1 needle)
1	5 ml syringe
1	10 ml syringe
1	20 ml syringe
1	25 g needle
1	28 g, 2 inch needle
1	#11 blade
1	#15 blade
1	surgical lubrication gel
	Dressing Supply
1	package of 4 × 4 gauze
1	sterile adhesive skin closure strips (Steri-Strips - 0.5 × 4 inch)
1	benzoin or Mastisol Adhesive Liquid
3	adhesive film dressing - medium (Tegaderm Transparent Dressing)
	Drugs Used in Sterile Field
	Marcaine 0.25% (without epinephrine) in a 10 ml syringe
	3.5–4.0 ml heparin 1000 units/ml in a 5 ml syringe
	saline in a 20 ml syringe

Planning Surgery Checklist

■ 1.   Choose a catheter for the patient.

■ 2.   With the patient's involvement, determine the optimum location for the catheter and mark the skin for the incision and exit site.

■ 3.   Choose a subcutaneous tunneler of the correct size and shape for making the subcutaneous exit path.

Preoperative Checklist

■ 1.   With the patient's involvement, review the location for the catheter and the marks that were made previously.

■ 2.   Give antibiotics to the patient.

Cefazolin 1000 mg IVPB

Alternatives: Vancomycin 500–1000 IVPB, Clindamycin 600 mg IVPB, Levofloxacin 500 mg IVPB

Operative Checklist

■   1.   Pause for the surgical team to go through and checkmark the instruments checklist and the safety checklist. Checklists covering all critical aspects are highly effective in contributing to positive outcomes and will be, in the future, the standard of care in all hospital operating rooms.

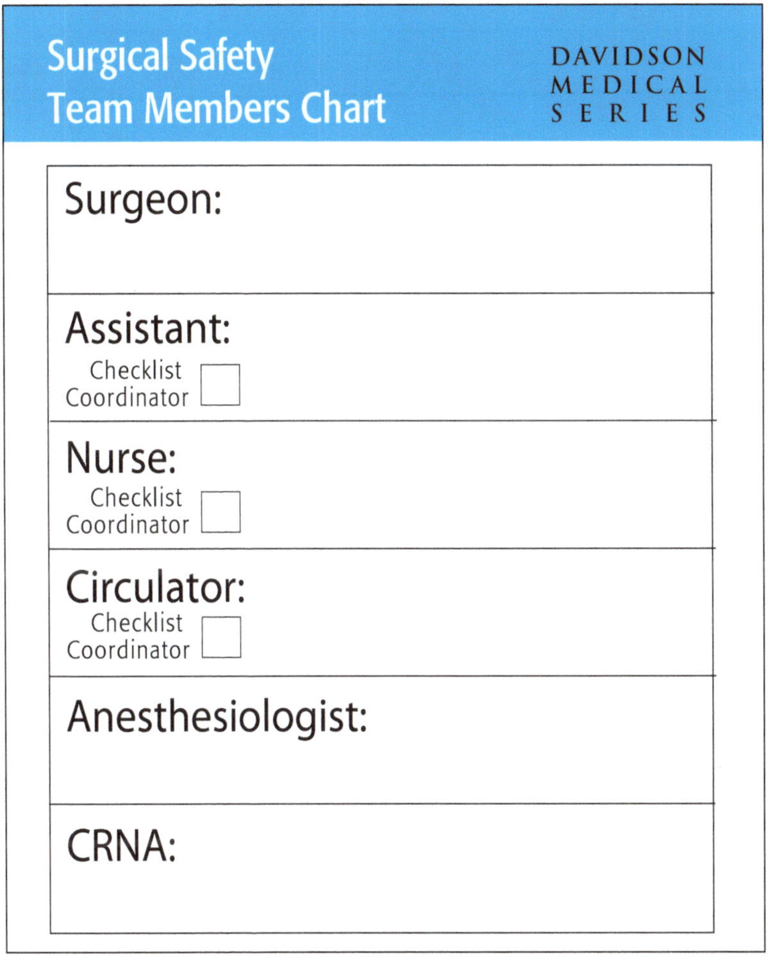

Surgical Safety Team Members Chart	DAVIDSON MEDICAL SERIES
Surgeon:	
Assistant: Checklist ☐ Coordinator	
Nurse: Checklist ☐ Coordinator	
Circulator: Checklist ☐ Coordinator	
Anesthesiologist:	
CRNA:	

Figure 3.1. Example of Surgical Safety: Team Members Chart

Surgical Safety
Patient Information

DAVIDSON
MEDICAL
SERIES

Name:			
Medical Record Number/ID:			
Diagnosis:			
Procedure:			
Dialysis Status			
☐ Not yet started			
☐ Current access Last dialysis date:			
Serum K:			
Pertinent Drugs			
Coumadin	☐ Yes	☐ No	
Plavix	☐ Yes	☐ No	
Beta blockers	☐ Yes	☐ No	
Others:			
List Allergies:			
1. 2.			
Have preoperative antibiotics been given? ☐ Yes ☐ No			
Is the incision, subcutaneous exit path, and exit site marked on the patient's body? ☐ Yes ☐ No			

Figure 3.2. Example Checklist for Surgical Safety: Patient Information

Instruments & Supplies Checklist
PD Catheter Placement - Open

DAVIDSON MEDICAL SERIES

Number In Set	Count at Sign In	Count at Sign Out	Surgical Instruments and Supplies
1			sterile marking pen
1			straight suture scissors
1			regular Metzenbaum scissors
1			fine Metzenbaum scissors
1			Allis forceps
1			tonsil hemostat
2			hemostat - curved
4			Mosquito hemostat - curved
2			Adson forceps - with teeth
2			DeBakey forceps
1			tissue forceps
1			Richardson retractor – baby or medium
1			Weitlaner retractor
1			Weitlaner retractor - baby
2			Senn retractors
1			US Army retractor
2			needle holder - regular
1			#3 knife handle
1			tunneling trocar (Blake Drain 15FR with Trocar – drain removed)
1			skin biopsy punch (optional)
1			stiff stylet for straightening the catheter
1			Tenckhoff catheter - 24'', 62.5 cm, 2 cuff
1			size 2-0 non-absorbable suture with ½ circle, taper point, 26 mm needle (Prolene Suture 2-0; SH needle)
1			size 5-0 absorbable suture with a ½ circle, taper point, 17 mm needle (PDS Suture 5-0; RB-1 needle)
1			5 ml syringe
1			10 ml syringe
1			20 ml syringe
1			25 g needle
1			28 g, 2 inch needle
1			#11 blade
1			#15 blade
1			surgical lubrication gel
			Dressing Supplies
1			package of 4 × 4 gauze
1			sterile adhesive skin closure strips (Steri-Strips - 0.5 × 4 inch)
1			benzoin or liquid adhesive (Mastisol Liquid Adhesive)
3			adhesive film dressing - medium (Tegaderm Transparent Dressing)
			Drugs Used in Sterile Field
			Marcaine 0.25% (without epinephrine) in a 10 ml syringe
			3.5–4.0 ml heparin 1000 units/ml in a 5 ml syringe
			saline in a 20 ml syringe

Figure 3.3. Example Instruments and Supplies Checklist for Open Placement of a Two Cuff, Coiled Catheter
The checklist has columns for checking items into and out of the operating room.

▪ 2.   Prepare the abdomen for surgery.

▪ 3.   Remark the skin (as need, to darken any faded marks) for the incision
        and catheter exit site.

        sterile marking pen

▪ 4.   Make the skin incision.

        #15 blade

▪ 5.   Dissect through the subcutaneous tissue to the anterior rectus muscle
        fascia. Maintain exact hemostasis.

        #15 blade
        electrocautery (setting; 20–25)
        mosquito hemostat
        tonsil hemostat
        Weitlaner retractor
        Senn retractor
        US Army retractor
        Metzenbaum fine scissors
        DeBakey forceps

▪ 6.   Incise the anterior rectus fascia; split the rectus muscle bluntly down
        to the posterior rectus fascia. Insert a retractor.

        Metzenbaum fine scissors
        Weitlaner retractor (alternatives: Senn retractor. US Army retractor)

▪ 7.   Place 1 or 2 tonsil (or Mosquito) hemostats to lift the fascia (and peri-
        toneum) up and away from the intra-abdominal contents. Using fine
        scissors, incise a small hole (3 mm) through the posterior rectus fascia
        and peritoneum, only large enough to facilitate the PD catheter inser-
        tion.

        tonsil or mosquito hemostats
        Metzenbaum fine scissors

▪ 8.   Place a purse-string suture around the small hole about 5 mm away
        using a 2-0 Prolene suture on a SH needle starting and ending above
        (cephelad) of the small peritoneal incision. To prevent the accidental

suturing of intra-abdominal structures, lift the peritoneum with a blunt instrument such as a curved hemostat.

Prolene Suture, 2-0, SH needle
curved hemostat

9. Prepare to insert the stiff stylet into the catheter by filling the catheter with saline. Insert the stylet while dripping wet gauze is held against the insertion end so that the catheter and stylet are continuously wetted; otherwise, the stylet may become stuck and be difficult to pull out. Sterile surgical lubrication gel greatly facilitates the stiff stylet insertion.

Tenckhoff PD catheter, 2 cuffs (62.5 cm long for most adults)
saline solution
stiffening stylet
surgical lubrication gel

10. Insert the catheter through the peritoneal opening. Let the catheter slide in. If resistance is encountered, back up and change direction. When the catheter is in 5 to 10 cm, retract the stylet somewhat which releases the coiled end. Place the now coiled end in the pelvic area.

11. Slowly remove the stylet with 1 hand holding the PD catheter in place at the exit site. Tie a purse-string suture snugly around the catheter.

Prolene Suture, 2-0, SH needle

12. The needle, still attached to the tied purse-string suture, is now placed through the back side of the peritoneal Dacron cuff and tied again. This locks the peritoneal cuff and catheter into place and keeps it from sliding up and down.

13. Test the flow function of the catheter by injecting 20–60 ml of saline into the catheter and aspirating gently or draining by gravity. Adjust the catheter placement until good drainage function is achieved.

20 ml syringe
saline

■ 14. Inject 0.25 % Marcaine (without epinephrine) to anesthetize the rec-
        tus muscle, fascia structures, and the subcutaneous tissue and tract.
        Inject into the wound to avoid contamination from skin bacteria.

        10 ml syringe
        Marcaine 0.25% (without epinephrine)

■ 15. While retracting the skin and subcutaneous tissue upwards exposing
        the anterior rectus fascia, use a mosquito hemostat to pull the catheter
        and the subcutaneous Dacron cuff through the anterior rectus fascia
        2–3 cm above the incision.

        US Army or Richardson retractor
        mosquito or right angle hemostat

■ 16. Attach the subcutaneous tunneler to the loose end of the catheter.
        From inside the incision site, penetrate just under the skin following
        the previously determined path, as marked on the skin. The subcuta-
        neous Dacron cuff is placed 1.5–2.0 cm inside the exit site. This usually
        requires some (digital) dissection.

        tunneling trocar (#15 Blake Drain or Faller Tunneler)
        skin biopsy punch (optional)

■ 17. Test the flow function of the catheter again by injecting 20–60 ml of
        saline into the catheter and aspirating gently or draining by gravity.
        Rapid, unobstructed drainage function must be achieved.

        20 ml syringe

■ 18. Gather the 3 occlusion pieces that come in the catheter kit: a clamp, a
        luer end piece, and a cap that screws onto the luer end piece. Insert the
        ridged or barbed end of the luer piece into the catheter tube. Insert the
        5 ml heparin syringe into the luer piece and inject 3.5–4.0 ml of hepa-
        rin (concentration 1000 units/ml) into the catheter to avoid catheter
        obstruction from blood clots. Leave the heparin syringe attached and
        clamp the tube midway with the catheter occlusion clamp to suspend
        the heparin in the catheter and prevent the heparin from leaking out
        the luer end or from flowing into the abdomen and defeating the pur-
        pose. Remove the 5 ml syringe and twist the cap into the luer insert.

        heparin 3.5–4.0 ml, 1000 units/ml

5 ml syringe
catheter luer end
catheter luer cap
catheter clamp

19. Close the anterior rectus fascia with a permanent suture, applied in a running or interrupted fashion, with tightly spaced stitches for a "watertight" seal.

Prolene Suture, 2-0, SH needle

20. Close the skin with 3–4 interrupted, inverted sutures using an absorbable suture; a running subcuticular suture may be added to complete the surgery.

PDS Suture, 5-0, RB-1 needle

21. Dressing the PD catheter wound involves several important steps. Suggested dressing material is pictured in Figure 2.48. Benzoin or Mastisol Adhesive Liquid helps to place a longitudinal, adhesive sterile closure strip on the incision (Figure 2.49). Place a folded, incised gauze around the catheter at the exit site (Figure 2.50). Place a second folded piece of gauze on top of the Steri-Strip (Figure 2.50). An extra layer of gauze will prevent the catheter and clamp from coming in contact with the skin (Figure 2.51). One or two adhesive film dressings are placed over the gauze, and the catheter is rolled up on top of the transparent film, making sure no catheter part or clamp is in contact with the skin (Figure 2.52). Place gauze over the rolled up catheter to facilitate removal and dressing changes (Figure 2.53). Place 2–3 adhesive film dressings over the gauze, taking care to avoid adhering the film to the catheter (Figure 2.54). One or two more transparent film dressings may be needed for a complete seal.

benzoin or Mastisol Liquid Adhesive
Steri-Strip 0.5 × 4 in/12 mm × 100 mm
Tegaderm Waterproof Transparent Dressing - medium size
gauze 4 × 4 in

LAPAROSCOPIC PLACEMENT
OF A TWO CUFF, COILED CATHETER

I   INSTRUMENTS CHECKLIST AND SURGICAL STEPS
II   LAPAROSCOPIC APPROACHES IN A HOSTILE ABDOMEN

I. DAVIDSON, C. HWANG, A. PARAMESH, D. SCOTT, D. SLAKEY

In this chapter, as throughout this publication and in the instructional video, placement of a straight neck, 2 cuff, coiled (62.5 cm) catheter is demonstrated.

Table 4.1. Instruments, Supplies, and Drugs for Laparoscopic Placement

Number In Set	Basic Instrumentation
1	Veress insufflation needle
1	laparoscopic camera, 5 mm, 30 degree
1	laparoscopic camera, 5 mm, 90 degree (optional)
1	5 mm VersaStep port or 5 mm Endo Tip Trocar with multifunctional valve
1	laparoscopic grasper
1	18 g, 3.5 inch spinal or 7–9 cm long, SDN disposable needle
1	22 Fr PTFE peel away introducer set
1	0.035 inch diameter guidewire
1	straight suture scissors
1	Adson forceps - with teeth
1	needle holder - regular
1	#3 knife handle
1	tunneling trocar (Blake Drain 15 FR with Trocar – drain removed)
1	3 mm skin biopsy punch (optional)
1	stiff stylet for straightening the catheter
1	Tenckhoff catheter - 24 inch, 62.5 cm, 2 cuff
1	absorbable suture with needle (PDS*II, 5-0, RB-1)
2	5 ml syringe
1	10 ml syringe
1	20 ml syringe
1	#11 blade
1	sterile surgical lubrication gel
	Dressing Supplies
1	package of 4 × 4 gauze
1	sterile adhesive skin closure strips (Steri-Strips - 0.5 × 4 inch)
1	benzoin or Mastisol Adhesive Liquid
4	adhesive film dressing - medium (Tegaderm Transparent Dressing)

continued on page 70

continued from page 69

	Drugs Used in Sterile Field
	saline in a 5 ml syringe
	Marcaine 0.25% (without epinephrine) in a 10 ml syringe
	3.5–4.0 ml heparin 1000 units/ml in a 5 ml syringe
	saline in a 20 ml syringe

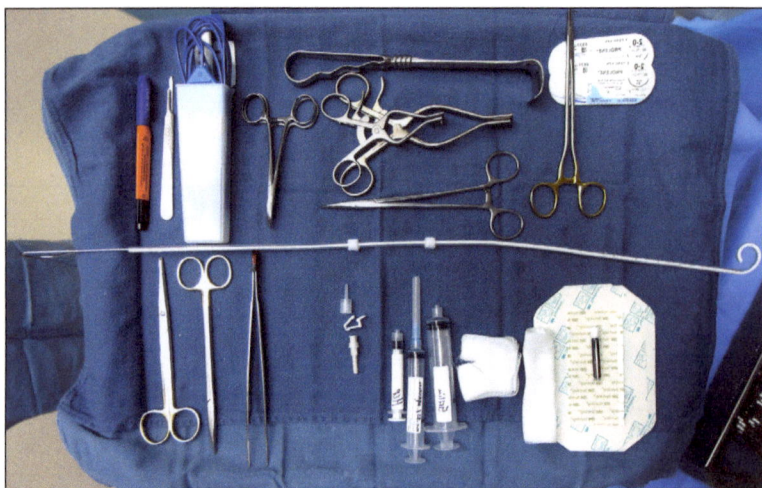

Figure 4.1. Basic Open Placement Instrument Tray

The instrument tray in Figure 4.1 (for open placement) is 1 of 2 trays used in the laparoscopic procedure for placing a 2-cuff PD catheter. This tray is an example of the author's approach to a consistent, efficient, and safe working environment, where instruments are kept in the same place at all times and in the order of initial anticipated use. This concept is consistent with what a commercial airline pilot expects and will indeed find every time he or she walks into the airplane cockpit. Instruments are lined up in the approximate anticipated order used. For detailed operative description of open catheter placement, see Chapter 2.

Figure 4.2 depicts examples of additional instruments used when the laparoscopic approach is chosen. For safety reasons the authors stress using syringes of different sizes for specific purposes (Figure 4.3) or even color-coded syringes to take safety one step further (Figure 4.4).

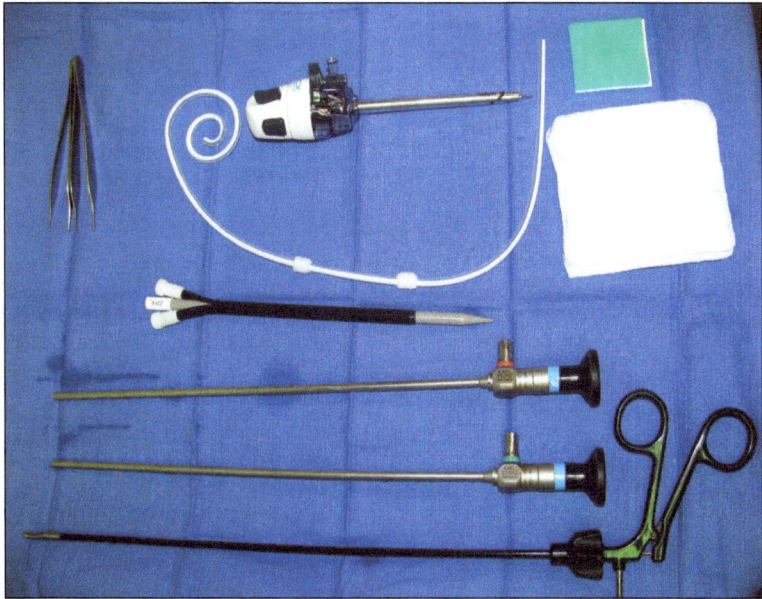

Figure 4.2. Laparoscopic Instrument Tray
A second operating room tray holds instrumentation specific to the laparoscopic procedure for catheter placement. Pictured upper left: Edson forceps with teeth; center from top: Endo Tip Trocar, 2 cuff, coiled catheter, peel-away dilator, 2 cameras, and a grasper; upper right: camera defogger and gauze.

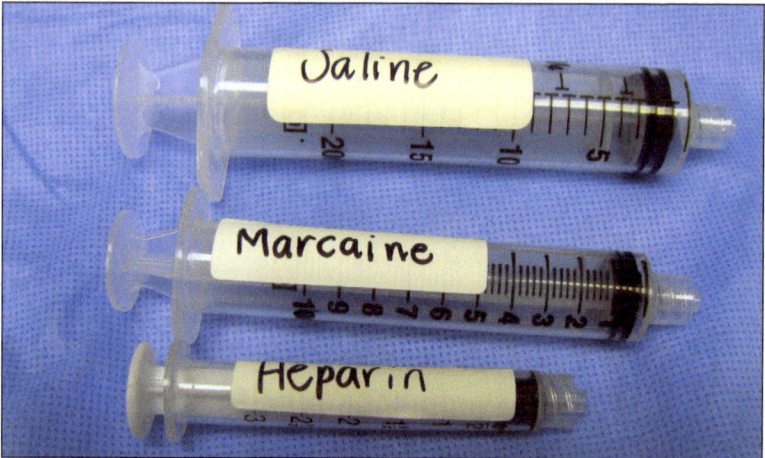

Figure 4.3. Syringes Labeled for Safety and Convenience
Injection syringes should be of different sizes, commensurate with the volume of drugs being served. For safety purposes and to avoid inadvertent use, each syringe is marked for content. The 5 ml syringe is for injecting heparin into the catheter at the end of the surgery. The 10 ml syringe is used to inject buvicaine (0.25% Marcaine) at the camera port incision, the catheter insertion incision, and into the rectus muscle during the creation of the extra-peritoneal tunnel. The 20 ml syringe is used for saline irrigation.

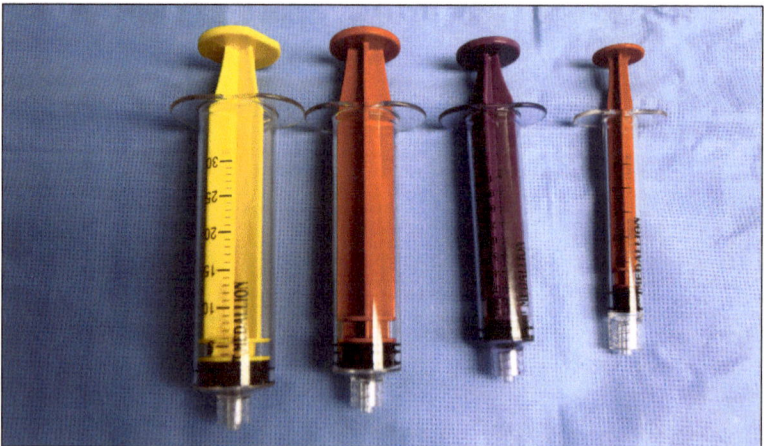

Figure 4.4. Color-coded Syringes
Using color-coded syringes advances safety one step further. When filled, the syringes must be marked for content. Hospitals are often reluctant to use these types of color-coded instruments and tools for policy and perhaps cost reasons.

GENERAL NOTES ABOUT OPEN VERSUS LAPAROSCOPIC PLACEMENT

PD catheters are typically inserted using either an open approach or a laparoscopic technique, dictated by the level of comfort of the operating surgeon, the patient's medical risk, and institutional resources. PD catheter placement using the blind Seldinger technique, under fluoroscopic guidance, and or under peritoneoscopic visualization are strongly discouraged because of increased risk of inadvertent visceral injury (1).

The open approach is associated with a shorter operating time and can be performed under spinal or local anesthesia, although general anesthesia is preferred (2,3–8). Laparoscopic placement requires general anesthesia, which may preclude some patients from undergoing placement. The laparoscopic approach makes it possible to perform additional indicated procedures under direct visualization including placement of the tip of the catheter and securing the tip of the catheter in the pelvis (6,8), as well as the ability to repair umbilical hernias with lysis of adhesions, and omentopexy (9–11). The open approach is more cost-effective, as only basic equipment is required for the procedure (3). Laparoscopy is the best technique to rescue problem catheters (9,10). Comparisons of open versus laparoscopic PD placement do not favor one technique over another (7). A thorough evaluation of the patient's suitability for PD, followed with mindful, patient-driven decisions and doing the *right* thing each time is likely to yield the overall best outcome for each patient. (Table 1.2)

The laparoscopic technique of PD catheter placement is discussed in detail in this chapter. The open technique is detailed in Chapter 2 and summarized in checklist format in Chapter 3.

PLANNING SURGERY STEPS

1. Choose a catheter for the patient. See Chapter 2 for details.

2. Determine the optimum location for the catheter and mark the skin. See Chapter 2 for general details about determining the optimum catheter location for each patient (Figure 4.5). As with the open placement, mark the skin with an indelible pen to indicate the catheter insertion incision, the subcutaneous path, and the exit site. For laparoscopic placement, additional marks are added for the costal margins, and the Veress needle/camera port(s). As a general rule, the insufflation needle should be 10–12 cm away from previous surgical scars. In patients with a previous cholecystectomy, the right subcostal area should be avoided. If a Hasson port is planned, a slightly larger inci-

sion must be made to assure access to a free peritoneal cavity and avoid visceral injury.

For patients with no previous abdominal operations, only 1 camera port incision is needed along with the catheter insertion site incision. This represents a significantly less invasive and more simplified procedure than the 2 instrument ports generally recommended. Incidental minor surgical procedures such as repair of small umbilical hernias and omentopexy can also be accomplished with only 1 port. More complicated and extensive laparoscopic repairs may require 1 or even 2 additional ports as described in Section II of this chapter.

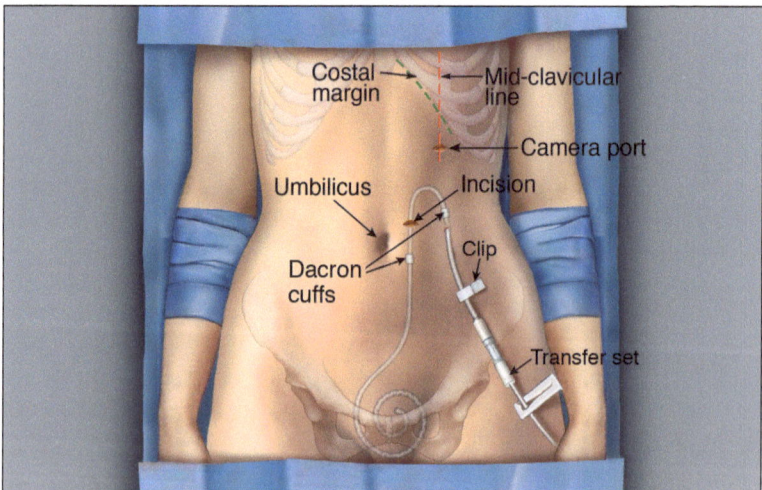

Fig 4.5. Surgical Anatomy in Relation to Laparoscopic Catheter Placement
Determining the size and location of incisions at the insertion site and port sites are crucial for successful laparoscopic placement and open placement.

3.   Choose a subcutaneous tunneler. See Chapter 2 for details.

General Notes about Anesthesia

Although laparoscopic placement of a PD catheter can be performed under local anesthesia and IV sedation, general anesthesia with a secure endotracheal airway intubation is safer and preferred for patient comfort. A LMA may not constitute a secure and safe airway, where changing the patient's position on the operating table is part of the procedure.

Supplemental local anesthesia 0.25–0.5% bupivacaine (Marcaine) in all dialysis access surgery induces a postoperative pain-free period of up to 12 hours, allowing the patient to reach home before needing additional oral pain medication.

Many patients undergoing dialysis access have uremic symptoms, with significant co-morbidity, most notably heart disease, hypertension, anemia, and diabetes. Dosing of anesthetic drugs must be decreased accordingly and given with great caution to avoid serious complications including intra-operative respiratory and circulatory arrest, and hypotension—not only jeopardizing the procedure itself but also inducing other complications such as strokes, cardiac events, or requirements for intubations and prolonged ventilator treatment. Individuals with HIV and Hepatitis C are candidates for epidural or general anesthesia to protect the operating room personnel from sudden movement in a sedated patient having a less than optimal regional block.

PREOPERATIVE CHECKLIST

1. With the patient's involvement, review the location for the catheter and the incision marks made previously. Remark any marks that may have faded.

2. Give the antibiotics—Cefazolin, 1 gram IV piggyback. In cases of allergy: Vancomycin 500 –1000 mg, Clindamycin 600 mg, or Levofloxacin 500 mg IV are alternative options for adults. In cases where it is not practical to give the antibiotics in the preoperative area, they can be given in the operating room, before the skin incision.

OPERATIVE STEPS

1. The surgical team pauses to verify the patient's name, medical record number or identification number, surgical side (right or left), incision site, and type of procedure. The surgeon briefs the team of any anticipated procedural deviations. Instruments and supplies are logged and checked into the operating room on the Instruments Checklist. Items listed on the Safety Checklists are checked off— Does the patient have allergies? Have antibiotics been given? See Chapter 3 for examples of Safety Checklists.

2. Prepare the abdomen for surgery—shave as needed, prep, and drape.

3. Remark the skin with a sterile, indelible marking pen to darken any marks that may have been removed during surgical prep. Mark the Veress needle site, camera-port site, catheter insertion site, and exit site.

    The surgeon usually stands on the patient's left side and the assistant on the right with 1 monitor on each side of the table at the patient's feet. The instrument table is on the surgeon's left side.

4. Using a #11 blade, make a 5 mm transverse skin incision to serve as the Veress needle insertion point and the 5 mm camera port.

    Use a tonsil hemostat to estimate the depth from the skin surface to the anterior fascia plane. Avoid spreading the subcutaneous tissues, as this will induce bleeding.

5. Insert the Veress needle, attached to a 10 ml syringe, straight in at a 90-degree angle. Resistance will be encountered at the depth measured with the hemostat. Two "pops" are felt as the needle penetrates the anterior and posterior muscle fascia planes. Aspirate for possible blood, bile, or "gas."

    Take the 10ml syringe off the Veress needle. With the syringe filled with saline, inject 1–2 ml into the Veress needle. As the syringe is removed again from the Veress needle, observe the fluid level fall in the needle as a sign of correct intra-abdominal needle location. This is known as the "drop-test."

6. Connect the CO_2 insufflation tubing to the Veress needle. Gradually start the CO_2 gas insufflation. Continue increasing pressure until the desired insufflation gas flow of 1.5–2.0 L/min until a pressure of 15 mm Hg is reached. If there is difficulty starting insufflation grasp the skin close to the Veress needle and lift the abdominal wall. Observe the abdomen. Percuss to assure accumulation in the intra-abdominal area. Remove the Veress needle when sufficient insufflation is obtained (12–15 mm Hg). Pressures above 15 mm Hg may compromise venous return.

7. Attach a 5 mm Endo Tip Trocar with multifunctional valves to the 90-degree camera (Figure 4.6). (The 90-degree camera is preferred for the initial view. For additional views of the anatomy and during the PD catheter insertion steps, a 30-degree camera is preferred.) Insert

the 5 mm Endo Tip trocar (Figure 4.7) into the abdomen and initiate camera vision to inspect the abdominal cavity for possible Veress needle injuries and incidental pathology. One can see the rectus muscle tissue as it is penetrated, and finally the posterior fascia and peritoneum before entering the abdomen.

Look for the presence of umbilical and inguinal hernias and other intra-abdominal pathology. Identify the inferior epigastric vessels. View the planned catheter insertion landmarks—away from the epigastric vessels and about 3 cm lateral to the midline, in this case the left side.

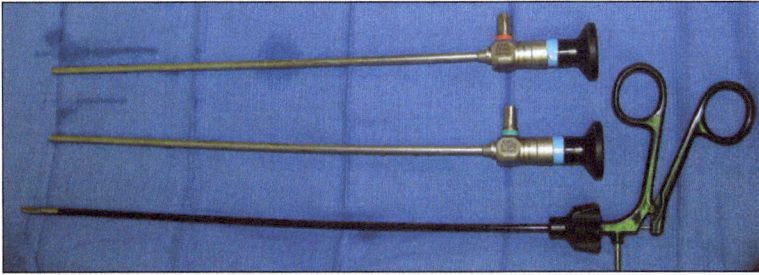

Figure 4.6. Two Cameras (30 degree and 90 degree) and Grasper

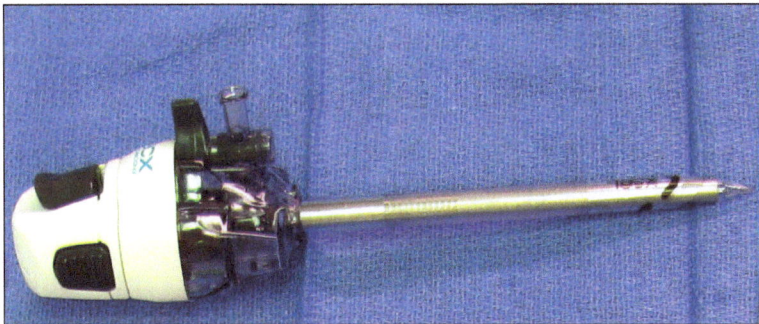

Figure 4.7. Endo Tip Trocar with Multifunctional Valve, 5 mm

8. Using a #11 blade, make a 5–7 mm transverse incision at the marked catheter insertion site. The incision is usually about 3 cm to the left of the midline and slightly above the level of the umbilicus (as is the case in this example).

A slightly larger skin incision is helpful when the catheter's sub-cutaneous cuff is later being pulled to the skin exit site.

9. Use a 10 ml syringe filled with 0.25% buvicaine (Marcaine) and attached to a disposable needle (18 g, 7–9 cm long) or a spinal needle—dictated by the degree of obesity. Insert the needle through the incision at the catheter insertion site, directed at an angle of about 45 degrees.

   As the needle is advanced along and between the peritoneum and the posterior rectus fascia for about 3–4 cm, Marcaine is injected between the peritoneum and the fascia to create a tunnel. The Marcaine will also provide postoperative pain control. The camera monitor shows the needle advancing, and a Marcaine-induced flare ridge, which represents the tunnel tract.

   Advance the needle until it penetrates the peritoneum, about 4–5 cm below the level of umbilicus and about 3 cm lateral to the midline in a downward angle of about 45 degrees. Remove the syringe, leaving the needle in place.

10. Insert the guidewire (0.35" DIA, 50 cm) into the peritoneal cavity, following the path of the needle. When the wire has reached the tip of the needle inside the peritoneal cavity, remove the needle.

11. Remove the peel-away sheath from the dilator (Figure 4.8). Insert the dilator over the guidewire using rotating movements. By first inserting just the dilator, the second pass, with the complete peel away set (Figure 4.9), is easier. The dilator is captured on intra-abdominal camera, going between the peritoneum and the posterior rectus fascia into the abdomen.

   Keeping the guidewire in place, remove the dilator and insert it into the peel-away sheath. The complete set—the dilator inside the peel away sheath—is now re-inserted over the guidewire into the abdomen using twisting movements, and guided by the intra-abdominal camera view. A small amount of sterile surgical lubrication applied to the outside of the peel-away sheath also greatly facilitates insertion into the abdomen. When the peel-away sheath is inside the abdominal cavity, the dilator is removed, leaving the sheath in place. At this point, a large amount of the pneumoperitoneum may be lost.

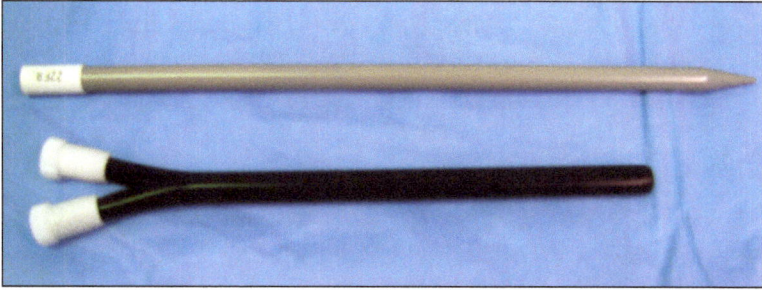

Figure 4.8. Introducer Set (22 Fr PTFE Peel Away Introducer Set, Cook)
Pictured on top: dilator; bottom: peel-away sheath

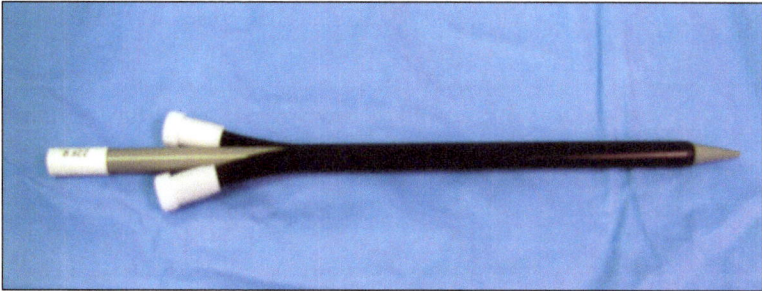

Figure 4.9. Introducer Set (22 Fr PTFE Peel Away Introducer Set, Cook)
The brown dilator is inserted into the black peel-away sheath.

12. Prepare the catheter by inserting a stiffening stylet to straighten the neck and the coiled segment. This step can be done in advance. For details on how to insert the stylet, see Chapter 2, step 9 and figures 2.16–2.19.

13. Insert the catheter (with the stiffening stylet inside) into the peel-away sheath that has been inserted into the patient's abdomen. Under camera vision, advance the catheter until the tip of the stiffening guidewire in the catheter is seen coming out of the sheath inside the abdomen. Pull the stiffening guide out enough to allow the coiled segment to recoil as the catheter is further advanced into the deep pelvic area. Continue to advance the catheter until the peritoneal Dacron cuff comes into view. Remove the stiffening guidewire. Remove the peel-away sheath by pulling and dividing the 2 external plastic limbs. Lodge the peritoneal Dacron cuff in its final position—either in the rectus muscle or at the level of the posterior rectus fascia—by grasping

the external portion of the catheter with 1 hand and pulling back. The position of the peritoneal cuff must take into consideration the correct placement the subcutaneous Dacron cuff, which rests 1.5–2.0 cm from skin level.

14. Attach the subcutaneous tunneler (Figure 4.10) to the external, free end of the catheter. By properly directing the tunneler, a smooth lumen will be formed as it tunnels subcutaneously along the marked path and exits through the skin. Insert the sharp tip under the edge of the incision and work the tunneler along the marked path through the subcutaneous tissue and out the exit site. Pull the tubing through the exit site until the subcutaneous Dacron cuff rests 1.5–2.0 cm inside the exit site. This usually requires some widening of the subcutaneous tissue tunnel with a hemostat. A snug fit between catheter and skin at the exit site will hold the subcutaneous cuff in place (Figure 4.11), making migration through the skin unlikely. The tunneler should exit the skin at an angle of about 30 to 45 degrees in order to optimize catheter-to-skin alignment and comfort for the patient. The exit site is ideally directed downward to keep the exit site clean and dry to help prevent infection. The cuff is placed at 1.5–2.0 cm from the skin.

No stitches should be placed at the exit site. Stitches create tension, which causes pain and trauma, promoting infection at the exit site. Also, when stitches have been placed, the patients sometimes think they are permanent and fail to return to have them removed.

Under no circumstances should a knife incision be made to force a hemostat retrograde to catch and pull the catheter out through the skin. This technique induces bleeding and can be quite traumatic to the skin, requiring stitches. The trauma and stitches cause complications and infection at the exit site. Because of their very sharp needlelike edge, tunnelers must be protected with a plastic cover (Figure 4.10) when not in use. Great care must be taken to avoid injuring operating room personnel. The surgeon should handle the subcutaneous tunneling steps with no help or interference from other team members.

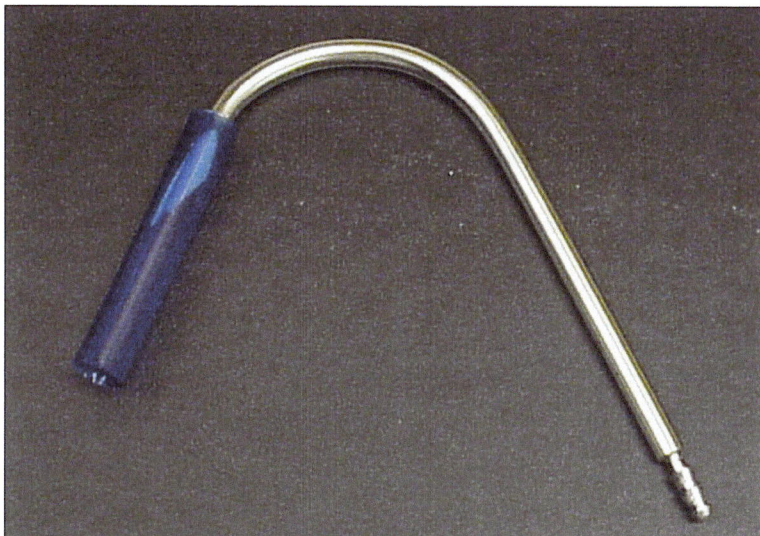

Figure 4.10. Blake 15 FR Tunneler
The authors prefer the 15 FR Blake drain tunneler with the plastic drain removed. The Blake tunneler is similar to the Faller tunneler except for the different blunt end with ridges that keep the catheter firmly attached while pulling through the tight skin at the exit site.

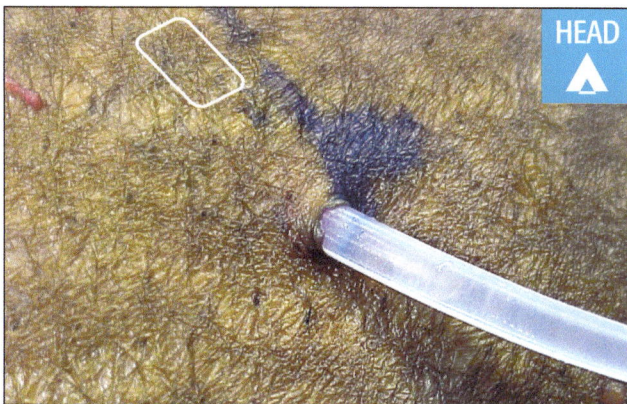

Figure 4.11. Detail of the Skin Exit Site
This close up image of the catheter exit site shows a snug fit with no bleeding, no stitches, and minimal trauma—thereby minimizing risk for postoperative infectious complications. The subcutaneous cuff is indicated by the white outline. The key to a snug fit is in choosing a tunneling device that is of the same or similar diameter as the catheter tube. It cannot be stressed enough, that stitches must NOT be placed at the exit site to "anchor" the catheter.

An alternative to puncturing the exit site with the tunneler from the inside is to use a skin biopsy punch (Figure 4.12 and 4.13). A 3 mm punch appears to be the ideal size as it creates a tight exit that fits snugly around the catheter. Care must be taken to advance the skin biopsy punch only through the dermis and epidermis as deep, maximal advancement may induce unnecessary bleeding.

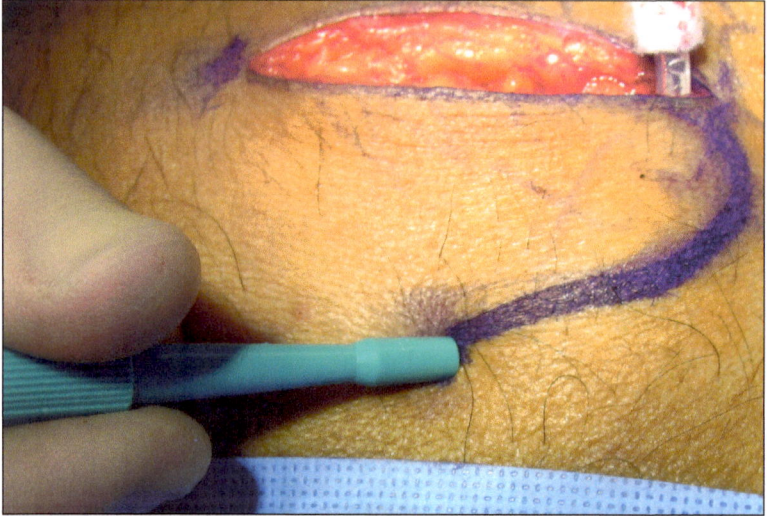

Figure 4.12. Skin Biopsy Punch Penetrating the Skin
Rotate the punch to gently to cut through the skin at an angle of about 45 degrees.

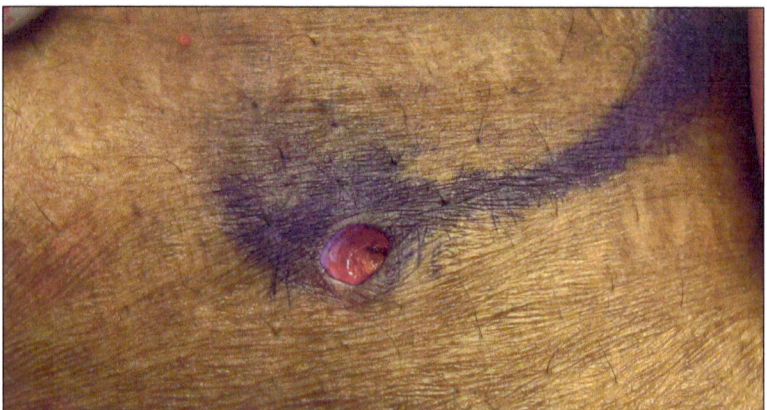

Figure 4.13. Completed Skin Biopsy Punch
The skin biopsy punch device creates a small lumen that fits snugly around the PD catheter.

15. Under camera view, using the 20 ml syringe, inject 20–60 ml of saline into the catheter and aspirate to rule out obstructions to flow, which at this point, can be confirmed by the return of CO_2 gas and fluid into the syringe. Also, it is recommended to test for obstructions by draining the catheter by gravity at the end of the case, after pneumoperitoneum has been removed. Rapid, unobstructed drainage function must be achieved. Leave 40–60 ml of saline in the abdomen in preparation for the next step. Should there be some blood in the abdomen, this can be irrigated through the PD catheter under direct camera vision. Using the camera, confirm that the coiled portion of the catheter is in position in the pelvis.

16. Gather the three occlusion pieces that come in the catheter kit: a luer end piece, a cap for the luer piece, and a clamp. Insert the ridged or barbed end of the luer piece into the end of the catheter tube with rotating movements while applying pressure on the luer piece. Insert the 5 ml syringe containing heparin into the luer piece and inject 3.5–4.0 ml of heparin (concentration 1000 units/ml) to prevent catheter obstruction from small blood clots or fibrin. The heparin now fills the 3.2 ml lumen volume of the 62.5 cm 2-cuff catheter, including the coiled portion. Leave the heparin syringe attached and clamp the tube midway with the catheter occlusion clamp to suspend the heparin in the catheter and prevent the heparin from leaking out the luer end or from flowing into the abdomen and defeating the purpose. The 40–60 ml of saline retained in the abdominal cavity in step 17 helps to suspend the heparin in the targeted areas. Remove the 5 ml syringe and twist the cap onto the luer insert.

17. With a 28 g, 2" injection needle, inject 0.25–0.5% Marcaine (without epinephrine) to anesthetize port site(s) and the catheter insertion site for postoperative pain relieve for up to 12 hours. Insert the needle into tissue inside of the wound to avoid contamination from skin bacteria.

18. Use the camera to assure that the coiled part of the catheter is deep in the pelvic area. Remove the camera.

19. Evacuate the CO_2 gas from the abdomen. Facilitate with gentle abdominal massage with the patient in a reverse Trendelenburg position.

20. Remove the Endo Tip Trocar.

■ 21. Close the skin incisions at the camera port site(s) and the catheter in-
        sertion site with 1 or 2 inverted sutures using a size 5-0 PDS Suture on
        a RB-1 needle.

        See Chapter 2, Step 21 for details about dressing the wounds and
        securing the catheter for the healing process.

II LAPAROSCOPIC APPROACHES IN THE HOSTILE ABDOMEN

Laparoscopic techniques can improve function of PD catheters (11). Patients
with ESRD who have had previous abdominal operations, including major
laparotomies are often turned down as candidates for PD catheter placement
because of the potential for complications. An initial laparoscopic evaluation
of the abdomen may indicate that PD is feasible, giving the patient at least
an attempt at PD. It is recommended to be prepared to place access for HD
in the PD operative setting should the PD attempt fail. With a laparoscopic
evaluation, the extent of adhesions and other pathology in the abdomen is
determined. Often the adhesions are minimal, allowing for concurrent PD
catheter placement and function. In other instances, a laparoscopic lysis of
adhesions will allow concurrent or delayed catheter placement. Another advantage of the laparoscopic placement of a PD catheter includes assessment of
the omentum. In cases where the omentum reaches the pelvis, omentopexy
may be performed to prevent catheter entrapment. Similarly, the catheter can
be sutured to the abdominal wall, in cases of catheter migration.

If laparoscopic placement is chosen, counsel the patient on the process,
explaining the possibility for needing a laparoscopic lysis of adhesions, or
even abandoning the procedure if the adhesions are severe. The side of placement may have to be determined in the operating room rather than preop-
eratively. The patient is informed that the catheter will likely be placed on the
side with fewer adhesions.

*The following steps are provided for cases where more extensive
laparoscopic surgery is called for.*

In place of Step 4

Make a 10 mm sub-umbilical transverse incision with a #11 blade large
enough to insert the Hasson trocar. This is usually the safest entry into an
abdomen with adhesions. Small S-retractors or US Army retractors are useful to visualize the midline fascia. Use 2 Kocher clamps to hold the fascia up
and minimize the risk of injury to other organs while incising the fascia with
a #11 blade.

In place of Step 5

Insert the 10 mm Hasson Trocar through the fascia defect, taking extreme care not to injure adhesion-engaged viscera. Once inside the peritoneal cavity, the Hassan trocar balloon is insufflated and Hassan stylet removed.

In place of Step 6

With the trocar attached to the CO_2 tubing, insufflate the abdomen to a pressure of 12–15 mm Hg, care taken to avoid unexpected high pressures or low CO_2 flow rates in the gas insufflation device caused by adhesions obstructing the flow of gas. A camera inserted into the trocar may help clarify the problem. Oftentimes, the trocar may need to be repositioned.

In place of Step 7

Insert a 90- or 30-degree camera through the 5 mm cap on the Hasson trocar to assess the extent of adhesions and the length of the omentum. Also, the amount of mesenteric fat and appendices epipoicae on the sigmoid is noted, as floppy and fatty sigmoid colon fat may wrap around and occlude the catheter. Based on these findings, the catheter may be inserted under laparoscopic visualization on the side found to have fewer adhesions.

Insertion of Additional Trocars

If adhesiolysis is deemed necessary, insertion of additional trocars will likely be required. A 5 mm incision is made infero-laterally to the umbilicus on the planned catheter insertion side. A 5 mm trocar is inserted through the rectus muscle under laparoscopic visualization. This will be the planned entrance site of the catheter into the peritoneum. A second 5 mm trocar may be inserted on the other side of the abdomen, to allow additional instrumentation and for rotation of optimal camera viewing during adhesiolysis. This second trocar is placed close to the first one, providing access for the grasper to guide the catheter through the planned entrance site.

Adhesiolysis is performed between the omentum/bowel and the anterior abdominal wall to create space and free the pelvic cavity. Adhesions in the upper abdomen should be left alone, as these help prevent the intestines and omentum from moving down into the pelvis, causing occlusion of the catheter (Figure 4.14). A combination of sharp dissection and cautery are used to divide the adhesions. Also, a pair of laparoscopic Metzenbaum scissors and a grasper are frequently utilized. A Kittner dissector is useful for gentle dissection and retraction.

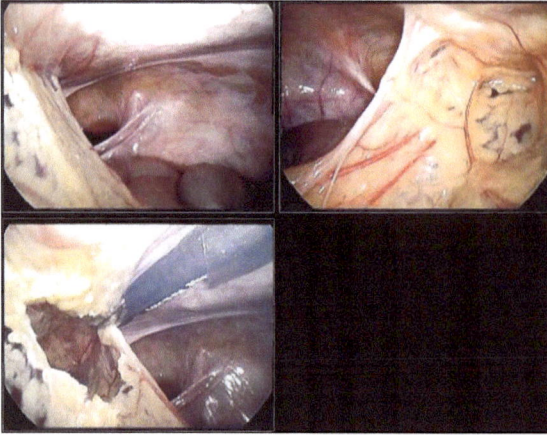

Figure 4.14. Detachment of Moderate Severe Adhesions

Moderate adhesions may be detached using a combination of laparo-scopic scissors, electrocautery, and a Kittner, dictated by the nature of the adhesion and the operator's discretion.

Careful attention must be paid to recognize and repair bowel serosal in-juries and tears, as patients with ESRD do not heal rapidly. Also, PD exchange fluids further impair healing.

Once the adhesiolysis is complete, the catheter is placed using the single 22 g peel-away dilator set, under direct camera vision, as described above in steps 8–13, in this chapter.

Alternatively, after the adhesiolysis procedure, the catheter can be placed as follows: With several ports in place, the grasper is passed from the lateral trocar (the second 5 mm trocar) through the planned insertion site (the first 5mm trocar), all the way to the outside of the body (Figure 4.15).

The insertion site trocar is then removed, leaving the grasper in place. This maneuver is necessary, as a catheter with cuffs will not pass through a 5 mm port. The tip of the catheter is held by the grasper and pulled into the peritoneal cavity and into the pelvis. The catheter is pulled up to a point where the peritoneal cuff lies just outside the peritoneum.

The rest of the insertion may proceed as previously described, con-tinuing with step 14. At the end of the procedure, the umbilical incision fas-cia is closed with interrupted suture in a "figure-of-8" fashion, ensuring a "watertight"seal.

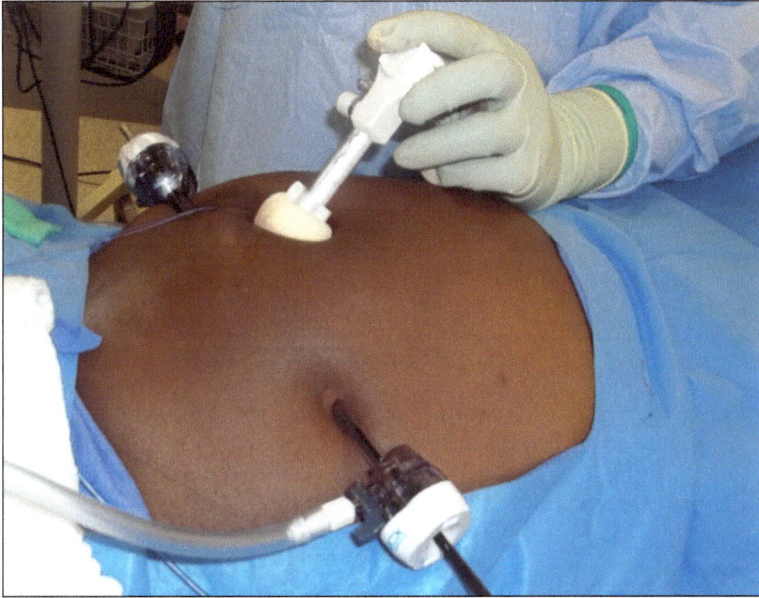

Figure 4.15. Alternative Catheter Placement
Ports may be added as indicated, based on intraoperative findings and required procedures.

Omentopexy is indicated during the time of initial laparoscopic insertion if the omentum reaches the pelvis enabling it to wrap around the catheter. Omentopexy can also be performed later, after an episode of omental occlusion. An Endostitch device (Ethicon) is inserted (Figure 4.16) through a 10 mm Hasson umbilical port to place a suture through the lowest part of the omentum. Alternatively, a grasper, inserted through a 5 mm port, pulls the omentum cephalad to the falciform ligament. Using the same suture, a second Endostitch bite is placed through the falciform ligament. The suture is then tied using the intra- or extracorporeal knot pusher technique. The omentum is elevated and attached to the falciform ligament. Further laparoscopic visualization should confirm that no part of the omentum will reach the pelvis.

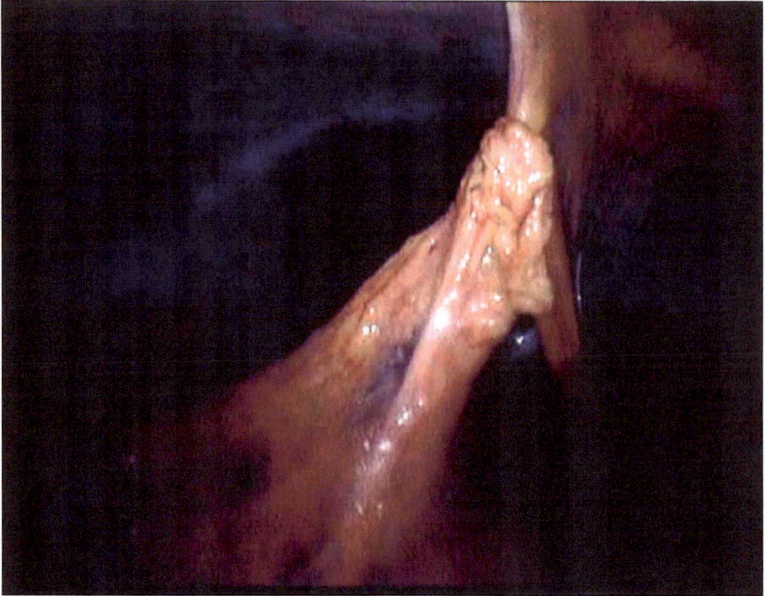

Figure 4.16. Laparoscopic Omentopexy
The omentum is lifted from the pelvis and sutured to the falciform ligament, using an Endostitch device.

For obstructed catheters and repeat migrations, the catheter can be stitched to the abdominal wall (Figure 4.17) with an Endostitch device (Ethicon) introduced through a 10 mm Hasson trocar at the umbilicus. A second 5 mm trocar camera port is placed in the upper abdomen. The catheter is mobilized and freed of any attachments to the omentum or mesentery and repositioned in the pelvis using a grasper inserted through the umbilical port. The Endostitch device is then introduced to make the first suture in the lower midline of the pelvis. The suture is then looped around the straight portion of the catheter and a second bite is taken next to the first suture. Another 5 mm trocar and grasper may be necessary to mobilize the catheter and help with looping the suture around it. A knot is then tied, aligning the straight portion of the catheter to the lower abdominal wall. (Figure 4.17) The knot must be tied loosely so as not to occlude the catheter lumen and to allow future removal. Care must also be taken to ensure that the straight portion of the catheter remains relatively opposed to the anterior abdominal wall to avoid internal hernias around redundant catheter loop.

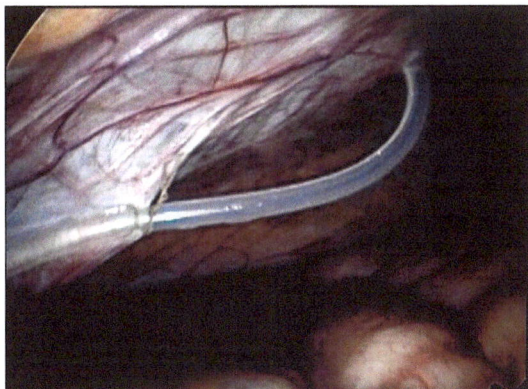

Figure 4.17. Example of Catheter Malposition
The catheter is sutured to the anterior abdominal wall.

Figure 4.17 depicts several important factors in catheter malposition. First, a permanent suture must be used such a polypropylene (Prolene Suture on a RB-1 or an SH needle). Second, the loop between the catheter entrance and the suture creates the potential for internal viscera hernia formation. Third, the catheter is entering the abdominal cavity at right angle, making it prone to migration. Proper alignment of the catheter—parallel to the anterior abdominal wall at the peritoneal entrance (emphasized in this publication and shown in Figures 2.22–2.28, 2.40)—largely prevents malposition of the intra-abdominal segment, as this alignment works with the catheter's "shape memory" or resilience force to maintain its position in the pelvis.

REFERENCES

1. Gadallah MF, Pervez A, El-Shahawy MA, et al. Peritoneoscopic versus surgical placement of peritoneal dialysis catheters: a prospective randomized study of outcome. *Am J Kidney Dis* 1999, 33: 118.

2. Maio R, FIgueiredo N, Costa P. Laparoscopic placement of Tenckhoff catheters for peritoneal dialysis: a safe, effective, and reproducible procedure. *Perit Dial Int* 2008. 28: 170.

3. Jwo SC, Chen KS, Lee CC, et al. Prospective randomized study for comparison of open surgery with laparoscopic-assisted placement of Tenckhoff peritoneal dialysis catheter – a single center experience and literature review. *J Surg Res* 2010, 159: 489.

4. Crabtree JH, Fishman A. Selective performance of prophylactic omentopexy during laparoscopic implantation of peritoneal dialysis catheters. *Surg Laparoscop Endoscop Percutan Tech* 2003, 13: 180.

5.   Dalgic A, Ersoy E, Anderson ME, et al. A novel minimally invasive technique for insertion of peritoneal dialysis catheter. *Surg Laparoscop Endoscop Percutan Tech* 2002, 12: 252.

6.   Tsimoyiannis ECT, Siakas P, Glantzounis G, et al. Laparoscopic placement of the Tenckhoff catheter for peritoneal dialysis. *Surg Laparoscop Endosc Percutan Tech* 2000, 10: 218.

7.   Wright MJ, Bel'eed K, Johnson BF, et al. Randomized prospective comparison of laparoscopic and open peritoneal dialysis catheter insertion. *Perit Dial Int* 1999, 19: 372.

8.   Santarelli S, Zeiler M, Marinelli R, et al. Videolaparoscopy as rescue therapy and placement of peritoneal dialysis catheters: a thirty-two case single centre experience. *Nephrol Dial Transplant* 2006, 21: 1348.

9.   Watson DI, Paterson D, Bannister K. Secure placement of peritoneal dialysis catheters using a laparoscopic technique. *Surg Laparosc Endosc* 1996, 6: 35.

10. Zadrozny D, Draczkowski T, Lichodziejewska-Niemierko K. Two-millimeter minisite mini-laparoscopy for rescue of dysfunctional continuous ambulatory peritoneal dialysis catheters. *Surg Laparosc Endosc Percutan Tech* 1999, 9: 369.

11. Attaluri V, Lebeis C, Brethauer S, et al. Advanced laparoscopic techniques significantly improve function of peritoneal dialysis catheters. *J Am Coll Surg* 2010, 211: 699.

CHARACTERISTICS OF AVAILABLE PERITONEAL DIALYSIS CATHETERS

Please refer to the "Appendix of Peritoneal Dialysis Products Cited in this Volume" for a list of companies that are holding copyrights or selling specific catheters cited in this chapter.

M. GALLIENI

For an optimal PD treatment, the availability of a well functioning PD catheter is of great importance, because characteristics of the PD catheter are related to incidence of peritonitis, efficiency of dialysis and to the overall quality of treatment. Indeed, PD catheter failure is responsible for dropout from PD in about 30% of cases (1). Table 5.1 lists the features of the ideal PD catheter.

It should be kept in mind that in addition to catheter features (materials, design), operator-dependent factors (implantation technique, catheter care) are also important aspects of good catheter function.

Table 5.1. Characteristics of the ideal PD catheter, which should enable simple, repeatable long-term access to the peritoneum.

Hydraulic function
- Optimal inflow and outflow (fast and complete draining of the peritoneal cavity)
- Largest possible internal diameter
- Kink resistant
- Design preventing obstruction
- No migration and displacement
- No fluid leakage

Biocompatibility
- No effect on physiology of abdominal tissues (body inert to catheter)
- No induction of inflammation, sclerosis, and adhesion of the peritoneal membrane

Resistance to infection
- Act as a barrier against microorganisms present at the exit site, preventing their entry into the subcutaneous tunnel
- Absence of factors favoring peritoneal infection (no biofilm, catheter resistant to bacteria and fungi)

Surgical handling
- Ease of implantation and removal

Patient friendliness
- Minimal interference with abdominal function and clothing
- Low cost

HISTORY OF PERITONEAL DIALYSIS CATHETER DEVELOPMENT

The lack of a safe method of accessing the peritoneal cavity, along with the development of a sterile technique, has been a major limiting factor in the diffusion of PD. In fact, the idea of treating uremic patients with fluids inserted in the peritoneal space dates back to 1923, when Georg Ganter at the University of Wuzburg treated a patient with infusions of 1500 ml saline solution. The patient initially improved, but died shortly thereafter (2)

Arthur Grollman (1901–1980) from Southwestern Medical School in Dallas developed a catheter that made PD treatment accessible for patients with ESRD using a 1-liter container with a cap that connected to plastic tubing (3). The tubing was then attached to a polyethylene catheter. The idea of using a flexible catheter design rather than a stiff tube, as had been the case in the past, was a great advance. In addition, Grollman added a new important feature to the catheter: several small holes in the distal part of the catheter. Inflow and especially the outflow of the dialysis solution were much improved.

In 1959, Maxwell et al (4) published a seminal paper, which assessed PD as a technique for the treatment of acute renal failure, describing access to the peritoneal space with a semi-rigid catheter. Weston and Roberts (5) devised a stylet catheter that could be readily introduced into the peritoneal cavity without a trocar. Only a small 6-French opening was made in the abdominal wall, which then stretched to fit the catheter so that little or no leakage occurred. Subsequently, the stylet catheter was also used for patients with CKD, but the necessity of repeated punctures represented a major problem. A permanent catheter would have allowed a better quality of life for patients and a wider acceptance of PD as a chronic dialysis technique. Palmer et al (6,7) reported the successful use of silicone rubber catheters designed to remain in place indefinitely. In 1968, Tenckhoff and Schechter (8) improved the PD catheter design by adding Dacron cuffs and developed a PD catheter that is still in use today. A flexible tubing made of silicone, has 1 or 2 cuffs which allow a firm adhesion to the tissues (the peritoneal cuff in proximity to and outside of the peritoneum membrane at the point of catheter entry into the peritoneal cavity, the subcutaneous cuff in proximity of the catheter exit site, or 1.5–2.0 cm from skin exit site), as well as reducing the possibility of tunnel infection and peritonitis (Figure 5.1).

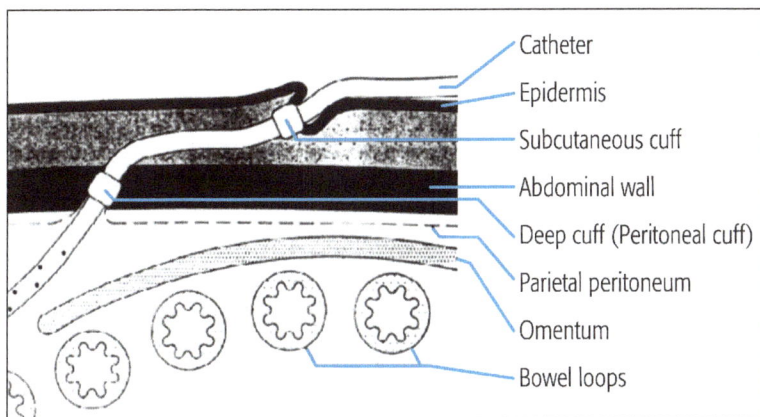

Figure 5.1. Schematic cut-away of a two-cuff Tenckhoff catheter in the abdomen, showing the position of the 2 cuffs.
(Ash S. *Int J Artif Organs* 2006; 29:85–94.) To make the figure consistent with terms used in this book, (Peritoneal cuff) has been inserted.

CURRENT USE OF PERITONEAL DIALYSIS CATHETERS

Catheter design and improvement is ongoing. This chapter examines and illustrates some of the commercially available products. Most of them are modifications of the Tenckhoff catheter (Table 5.2).

Negoi et al (9) assessed preferences in catheter design and implantation technique in 2004 from an international sample of 65 respondent chronic PD centers (Table 5.3). Figure 5.2 compares these numbers with a previous assessment in 1994 (9), showing an unchanged situation. In both adult and pediatric programs, the Tenckhoff catheter remains the most widely used catheter, although use of a pre-curved (swan neck) catheter is increasing. Double-cuff catheters continue to be preferred over single-cuff catheters, and coiled intra-abdominal segments are generally preferred over straight intra-abdominal segments (Figures 5.3 and 5.4). In most programs (75% of adult centers and 69% of pediatric centers), only 1 type of catheter is used and the surgical implantation technique remains the prevailing placement method (9).

TABLE 5.2. Commonly used Peritoneal Catheters

Tenckhoff and Tenckhoff-modified
Straight
  • Classic Tenckhoff
  • With inner discs (Oreopoulos-Zellerman, Toronto Western Hospital,)
  • Short (Vicenza)
  • Self-locating, with tungsten weight (Di Paolo)
Coiled
  • Tenckhoff
T-fluted (Ash Advantage)
Balloon (Valli)

Permanent bend
Swan-neck (permanent 150-degree arc)
  • Swan Neck Tenckhoff straight and coiled
  • Swan Neck Missouri straight and coiled
  • Moncrief–Popovich catheter
  • Pre-sternal, swan-neck catheter
Pail-handle (Cruz)

Continuous flow

Table 5.3. Distribution of Types of Catheters Implanted

Catheter type	Percent distribution
Tenckhoff, 2 cuffs, straight or coiled	60.7%
Swan Neck Tenckhoff, 2 cuffs, straight or coiled	18.0%
Swan Neck Missouri, 2 cuffs, straight or coiled	4.7%
Tenckhoff, single cuff, straight or coiled	4.0%
Toronto Western Hospital	4.0%
Cruz, 2 cuffs, coiled	2.6%
Pre-sternal, swan-neck, 3 cuffs, coiled	1.5%
Others	4.5%

The main types of PD catheters implanted in incident patients (n. 1102), according to a 2004 survey. Coiled catheters represented over 80% of cases. (Negoi D, Prowant BF, Twardowski ZJ. Current trends in the use of peritoneal dialysis catheters. *Adv Perit Dial* 2006; 22:147-52)

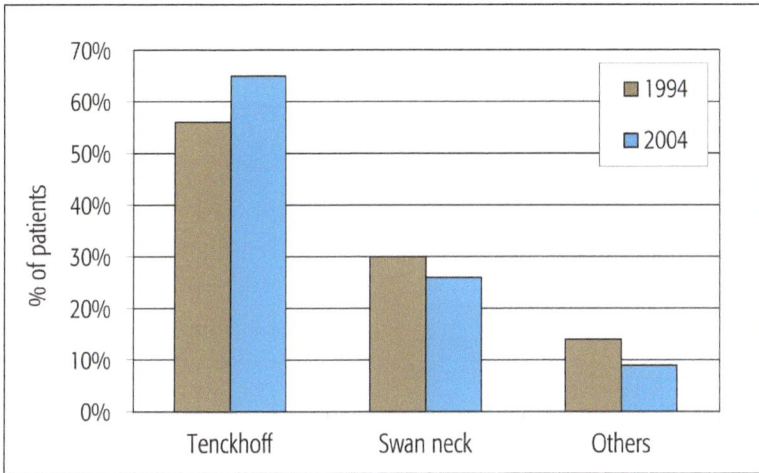

Figure 5.2. Percentage of Patients with Tenckhoff, Swan Neck, and Other Types of Catheters in 1994 and 2004 Surveys
A 2004 survey showed that the Tenckhoff catheter was used most often, with the Swan Neck catheter being the next most popular. These results are similar to those from a previous survey conducted in 1994. (Negoi D, Prowant BF, Twardowski ZJ. Current trends in the use of peritoneal dialysis catheters. *Adv Perit Dial* 2006; 22:147-52)

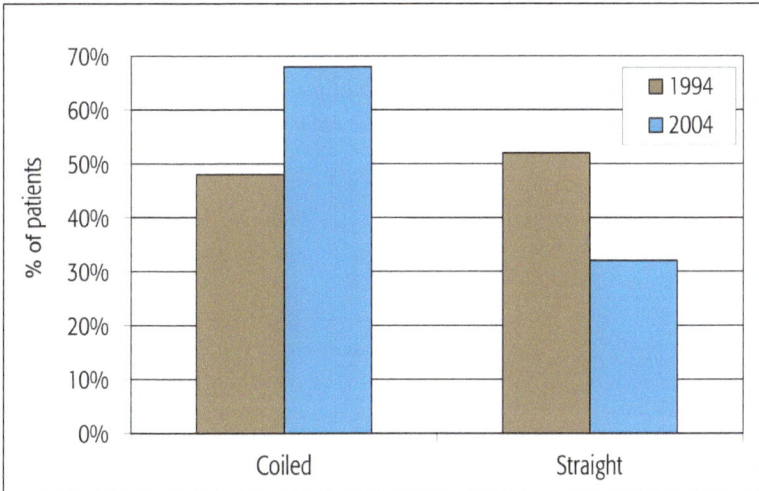

Figure 5.3. Catheters with coiled intra-abdominal segments are preferred for adult patients; with a 20% increase from 1994 to 2004.
(Negoi D, Prowant BF, Twardowski ZJ. Current trends in the use of peritoneal dialysis catheters. *Adv Perit Dial* 2006; 22:147-52)

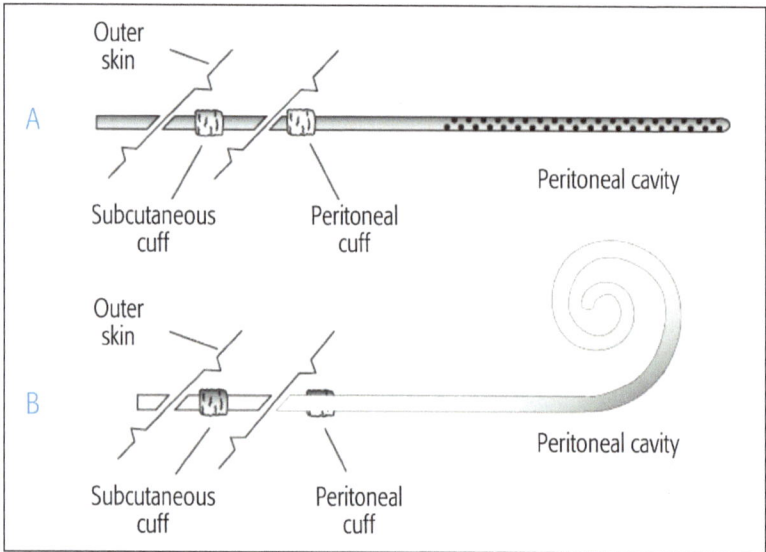

Figure 5.4. Straight (A) and Coiled (B) Tenckhoff PD Catheters
(NIDDK booklet "Treatment Methods for Kidney Failure: Peritoneal Dialysis" http://kidney.niddk.nih.gov/kudiseases/pubs/peritoneal/, accessed 9/4/2011)

CATHETER DESIGN AND DIALYSATE FLOW

In the design of a PD catheter, of utmost importance is consideration of an effective dialysate flow. Flow is dependent on the pressure gradient across the catheter and its hydraulic resistance (10). **Flow = Pressure/Resistance**

During inflow, the pressure gradient is established by the vertical distance between the dialysate bag and the intra-abdominal catheter tip. Likewise, during outflow, the pressure gradient is established by the vertical distance between the catheter and the drain bag. The flow rate can be increased by increasing the vertical distance between bags and catheter tip. In addition, the hydraulic resistance to flow is influenced by catheter characteristics, mainly its inner diameter. However, reducing the width of the catheter wall to achieve a larger diameter can predispose the catheter to kinking, unless a more resistant material than silicone is used.

Adult PD catheters have an outer diameter of approximately 5 mm, but there are three possible internal diameters:
- 2.6 mm is the standard internal size of the Tenckhoff catheter, Swan Neck catheter, Missouri Swan Neck catheter, and Toronto Western Hospital catheter
- 3.1 mm is the internal diameter of the pail handle (Cruz) catheter

- 3.5 mm, the largest internal diameter, can be found in Flex-Neck catheters and Ash Advantage catheters.

Fabrication Materials

Only 2 materials have been used successfully in the manufacture of PD catheters. Silicone is the most commonly used material, because of its good biocompatibility. Polyurethane has been introduced because it allows a thinner catheter wall, although some problems with its durability have been reported (see below "Pail-handle (Cruz) catheter" for further details).

Catheters with a Straight Intra-abdominal Segment

The classic Tenckhoff PD catheter (Figure 5.5) is easy to place by either percutaneous or surgical technique. It is also easy to remove and replace. When inserted, the Tenckhoff catheter can be considered as having three parts: 1. intra-abdominal; 2. subcutaneous tunnel; 3. external (Figure 5.1). The intra-abdominal segment has multiple small holes and an open terminal end. The subcutaneous segment has 2 cuffs. The subcutaneous cuff is placed 1.5–2.0 cm under the skin at the exit site, and the peritoneal cuff is placed just external to the fascia covering the parietal peritoneum. The segment between the 2 cuffs lies in a tunnel, classically curved in shape, and runs from the skin exit site to the peritoneal cuff.

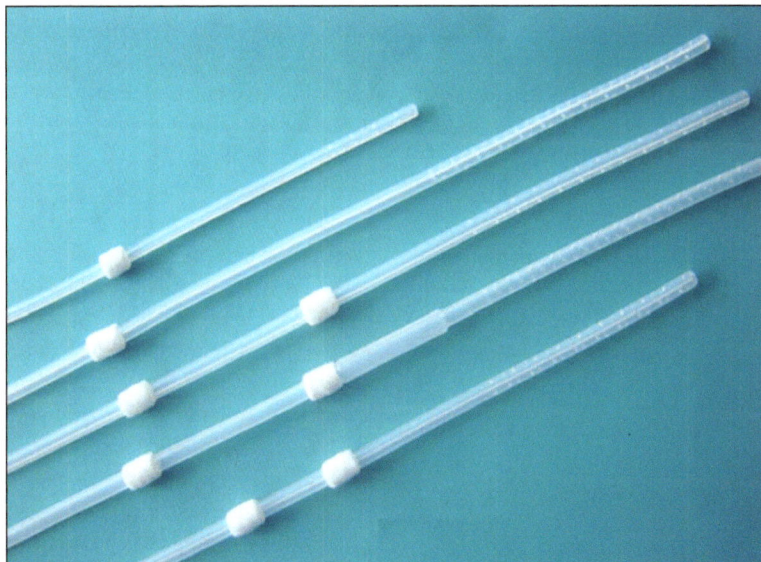

Figure 5.5. Tenckhoff PD Catheters with Straight Intra-abdominal and Subcutaneous Segments

Catheters with a Coiled Intra-abdominal Segment

The Coiled Tenckhoff catheter (Figure 5.6) has similar characteristics to the straight catheter, but is considered to have better patency and better outflow. It is also better tolerated because of a smoother contact with the pelvic organs. The intra-abdominal coiled configuration has been adopted by several other catheter models.

Despite the increasing number of implanted coiled catheters, in a systematic review of randomized controlled trials, straight and coiled intra-abdominal segments were found to be associated with similar rates of peritonitis, infection at the exit site and in the tunnel, as well as similar rates of catheter removal and replacement events (11). In addition, a small randomized study comparing straight and Short (Vicenza) coiled Tenckhoff catheters found a significantly higher frequency of flow problems due to malposition of straight catheters, requiring replacement of the catheter using a coiled catheter (12).

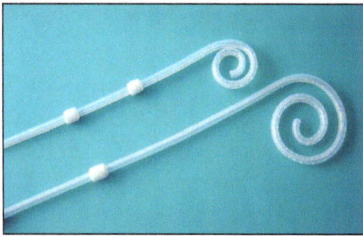

Figure 5.6. Coiled Tenckhoff PD Catheter

Permanently Bent Catheters

Swan Neck catheters (Figure 5.7) have a pre-formed 150° arc in the subcutaneous segment, designed to keep both the intra-abdominal and external portions of the catheter positioned downward. They are intended to keep the intra-abdominal portion from migrating out of position and to decrease stress on the exit site by the external portion, which often occurs when a straight catheter is manually curved during placement (13).

The Toronto Western Hospital catheters (Figure 5.8), also known as Swan Neck Oreopoulos-Zellerman, have a swan-neck configuration, but differ from other catheters in that 2 silicone discs are added to the intra-abdominal segment. The discs are designed to prevent omental wrapping, while keeping the catheter tip in the pelvis.

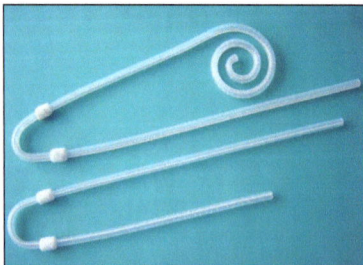

Figure 5.7. Swan Neck PD Catheters, Straight and Coiled Intra-abdominal Segments

In a single-center retrospective study of 208 Toronto Western Hospital PD catheters, Sikaneta et al (14) found catheter survival rates and complications rates similar to those reported in the literature for other peritoneal catheters.

The Missouri catheters (Figure 5.9) have the same basic design of a Swan Neck catheter, but the peritoneal cuff has a peculiar configuration, with the addition of a silicone bead and a polyester disk (15). The bead rests just inside the peritoneum to pre-

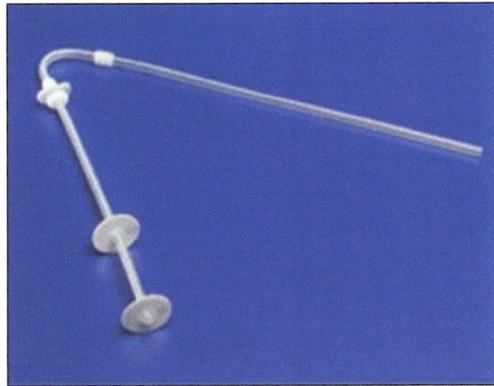

Figure 5.8. Swan Neck Toronto Western Hospital PD Catheter, Straight Intra-abdominal Segment

vent dialysate leakage. The felt disk is placed just outside the peritoneum and is sutured to the rectus muscle. This catheter has been suggested for patients who experience dialysate leakage; and due to its characteristics, it can only be placed and manipulated surgically. It is available with a straight or coiled intra-abdominal segment, as well as a presternal configuration (16) (Figure 5.9).

The Moncrief-Popovich peritoneal catheter has a swan-neck configuration and it is used in combination with the buried insertion technique (17). The larger 2.5 cm subcutaneous cuff, which is buried in the subcu-

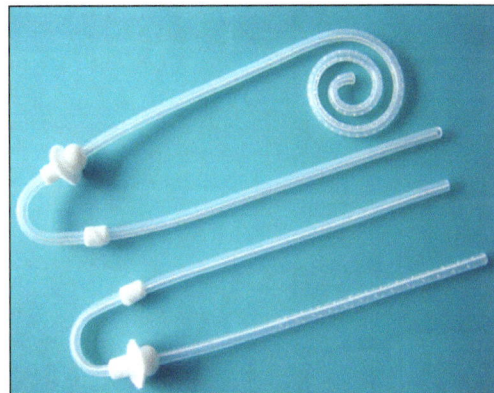

Figure 5.9. Swan Neck Missouri PD Catheter, Straight and Coiled Intra-abdominal Segments

taneous tissue for 3 to 6 weeks, is easier to locate when the external part of the catheter is recovered for the start of dialysis (18).

It has been proposed that this design should lessen catheter related complications, including peritonitis, tunnel/cuff infections, and leakage, by formation of an improved bacteriological barrier and maximum tissue ingrowth into the catheter cuffs in a sterile environment (19).

The Swan Neck Sendai catheter has a swan-neck configuration, but the subcutaneous cuff has a different position. It is inserted at the top part of the permanent bend (20). The subcutaneous cuff is anchored with 2 stitches of silk thread to the anterior rectus sheath to maintain the inverted U shape. According to Ishizaki et al (20), no break-in period is necessary and dialysis treatment sessions can be started immediately after the implantation of this catheter.

The Pre-sternal catheter (Figure 5.10), introduced into clinical practice 20 years ago (21), has a swan-neck configuration, with the exit site located on the anterior chest wall. A long tunneled segment with a swan-neck configuration connects to a standard straight or coiled Tenckhoff catheter. The 2 segments of the catheter are joined by a titanium connector at the time of implantation. The presternal location was conceived to reduce the incidence of exit-site infections compared to PD catheters with abdominal exits. Compared with abdominal catheters, dialysis-solution flow is slightly slower because of the increased catheter length. There is a possibility of catheter disconnection in the tunnel, but this complication is extremely rare in adults. Finally, the implantation technique is more challenging compared with that of single-piece, abdominal catheters.

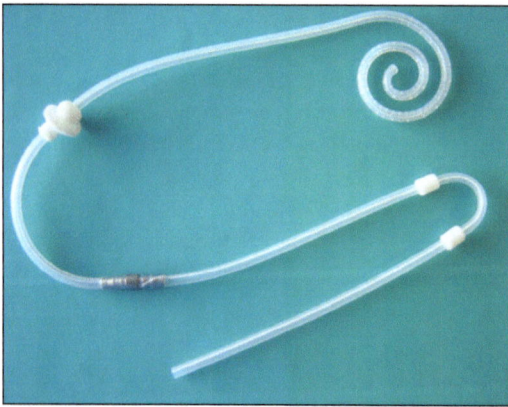

Figure 5.10. Swan Neck Pre-sternal PD Catheter, Coiled Intra-abdominal Segment

The presternal catheter is particularly useful in obese patients, in patients with abdominal stomas, urinary diversion, a higher tendency to exit-site infections, and in children (22). Some patients prefer the presternal catheter because of better body image and the possibility to take baths if the catheter exit site can be kept above water.

The Pail-handle (Cruz) catheter is peculiar for its shape and material. It is made with polyurethane, which makes a stronger and thinner catheter wall than silicone, while providing a larger inner diameter, and therefore more rapid inflow and outflow of the dialysis fluid (23). However, hydrolysis of the polyurethane surface apparently takes place. Cracking of the material with constant use has been reported, especially in long-lasting catheters when polyethylene glycol or alcohol is applied (24,25).

Another specific characteristic of this catheter is its 2 permanent right-angle bends: 1 to direct the intra-abdominal portion parallel to the parietal peritoneum, and 1 to direct the subcutaneous portion downward toward the skin exit site.

Modified Straight Catheters

Several modifications of the inner part of a classic straight Tenckhoff catheter have been proposed, including the T-fluted (Ash Advantage), balloon (Valli), short (Vicenza), and the self-locating catheter (Di Paolo).

The T-fluted (Ash Advantage) catheter. (Figure 5.11) is a T-shaped peritoneal catheter with a single transabdominal tube joining to a tube lying against the parietal peritoneum (26). Segments with long flutes (grooves) serve as fluid ports rather than the classic 1-mm diameter holes. The folded catheter is placed with a procedure similar to the one for a conventional Tenckhoff catheter, but once inside the peritoneal space, the flutes open into position adjacent to the parietal peritoneum and perpendicular to the transrectal portion. Outflow rate for the Ash T-fluted Advantage catheters has been reported to be about 30% higher than for Tenckhoff catheters, with outflow completed in 6 to 15 minutes. Catheter survival was 90% at 12 months. The catheter may be an alternative to conventional Tenckhoff catheters in patients at high risk of catheter failure.

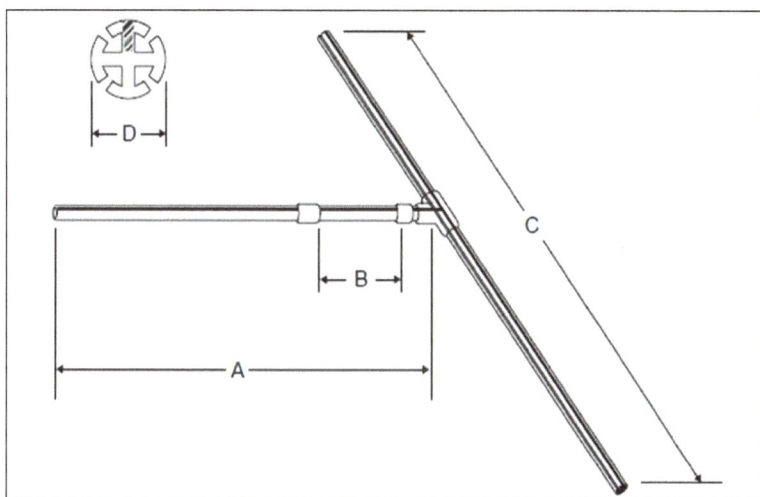

Figure 5.11. T-fluted Ash Advantage PD Catheter
Abbreviations: A: transabdominal tube length; B: distance between cuffs; C: overall intra-abdominal length; D: flute diameter.

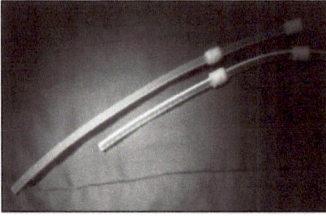

Figure 5.12. Short (Vicenza) PD Catheter

The Vicenza PD catheter has a shorter intra-abdominal segment, compared to a standard Tenckhoff catheter. (Dell'Aquila R, Chiaramonte S, Rodighiero MO, et al. The Vicenza "Short" peritoneal catheter: A twenty-year experience. *Int J Artif Organs* 2006; 29: 123-127)

The Balloon (Valli) catheter allows higher flow rates and presents lower fluid outflow problems compared to the standard Tenckhoff catheter. The main feature of this catheter consists in a perforated silastic balloon, which protects the distal end of a standard Tenckhoff catheter (27). It is rarely used.

The Short (Vicenza) catheter (Figure 5.12) is defined "short" as it consists of a classic straight double-cuff PD catheter with a much shorter intra-abdominal segment, compared to other catheters. It is implanted in the lower abdomen, between the navel and the pubis. In a publication by Vicenza (28), survival rates with the device at 2 and 5 years of 94.3% and 91.5%, respectively, have been reported. Due to its lower implantation site, this catheter demonstrated less dislocation and has excellent body image acceptance.

The self-locating (Di Paolo) catheter (Figure 5.13) counters the main disadvantage of the Tenckhoff catheter—the tendency for dislocation of the catheter tip (29,30). The degree of dislocation may be small—with the tip remaining in the lowermost part of the abdominal cavity, or large—with the tip migrating into the upper abdomen. Dislocation is among the most

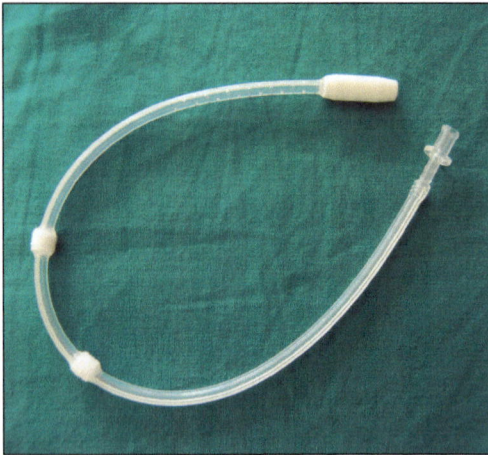

Figure 5.13. Self-locating (Di Paolo) Peritoneal Dialysis Catheter

The tip of the catheter has a heavy tungsten ring encased in silicone, preventing the catheter from floating on top of the dialysis fluid and maintaining it in the lower abdomen. (Di Paolo N, Petrini G, Garosi G, Buoncristiani U, Berardi S, Monaci G. A new self-locating peritoneal catheter. *Perit Dial Int* 1996; 16:623–7)

frequent reasons for catheter removal or substitution, as well as for dropout from PD.

The self-locating catheter was designed to avoid dislocation (31,32). Its main feature is the presence of a heavy tip, obtained by the insertion of 12 grams of silicone-encased tungsten, a physically and chemically inert element. The heavy tip prevents the catheter from floating on top of the dialysis fluid, keeping it in the lower abdomen. The catheter retains the classic Tenckhoff form with the same internal diameter. In the final 2 cm, the external diameter is slightly larger and the usual perforations are absent.

In most patients, the catheter is well tolerated, but in a few cases, especially women, some discomfort has been reported in the first days after catheter placement, possibly because of the contact between the catheter tip and the peritoneal membrane in the pelvic area. The discomfort diminishes and finally disappears with time and can be attenuated by leaving 200 to 500 ml of icodextrin in the peritoneal cavity.

A multicenter observational study (33) of 962 patients (746 self-locating and 216 Tenckhoff catheters) determined that patients with the self-locating catheter had fewer episodes of catheter displacement (0.8% versus 12% respectively). Duration of the self-locating catheter was significantly better, with a possible influence on dropout from PD. At the end of 2 years of observation, dropout was 38.4% for the Tenckhoff group and 22.0% for the self-locating group. In addition, patients with the self-locating catheter also showed fewer episodes of peritonitis, tunnel infection, cuff extrusion, catheter malfunction, obstruction, and leakage, compared to the traditional Tenckhoff catheter. These results are particularly interesting because up to the year of publication of this paper in 2004 (33), the major guidelines and a systematic review (11) indicated that no catheter seemed to be superior to the standard 2-cuff Tenckhoff catheter in the prevention of peritonitis, peritonitis rate, exit-site/tunnel infection rate, and technique failure.

Some concern has been expressed about the risk of abdominal magnetic resonance tests in patients with the self-locating catheter, due to the possible presence of ferrous impurities in the tungsten. Although it has been regarded as improbable (33), it should be kept in mind because there are no published studies that address this potential problem. When necessary, MR should be done with the peritoneal cavity full of fluid, which eliminates possible vibrations of the tungsten tip in the magnetic field.

Reinforced Catheters

Reinforced catheters are designed with an additional mass of silicone in the intra-abdominal segment, in order to prevent catheter dislocation from the pelvis. The reinforcement is made of the same implant-grade silicone as the catheter. They are available with straight or coiled intra-abdominal segments and straight or swan-neck subcutaneous segments.

Catheters for Children with Chronic Kidney Disease

Evaluation of PD for children with CKD follows criteria that are different from criteria for adults. Pediatric patients are heterogeneous, because their age ranges from days to 18 years, and their body weight between 2 and 50 kg. The adult catheter is used in children who weigh over 30 kg and a pediatric size is used in those below 30 kg. A neonatal catheter is available for use in infants under 5 kg body weight.

In children, the intra-abdominal length is very important. To achieve proper drainage, the catheter tip should lie in the child's pelvis. Neonatal catheters usually have a shorter, 5 cm tract of drainage holes but otherwise they are similar to pediatric catheters.

Initially, single-cuff Tenckhoff catheters were preferred (34,35), because they are easier to insert and to remove, a useful feature considering that a kidney transplant is often possible within a short time. However, this approach has changed over time. In a non-randomized controlled study, Lewis et al (36) found that peritonitis-related catheter loss was significantly more common with single-cuff catheters. The relative risk of staphylococcus aureus peritonitis with a single cuff compared to a double-cuff catheter was 2.1, and the relative risk of catheter loss with peritonitis was 7.5 for single-cuff catheters. They concluded that double-cuff peritoneal catheters are more effective than single-cuff catheters in preventing penetrating infection in infants and children. In 1998, in contrast to the situation in North America, the Italian registry (37) documented an 82.5% use of double-cuff catheters in children; and the North American Pediatric Renal Transplant Cooperative Study showed an increase in the use of double-cuff catheters to 34% in 1997 from 29.9% in 1993 (38). In the same report, it was also suggested that pediatric patients should be treated with PD catheters that have a swan-neck design, 2 cuffs, and downward pointing exit sites (38). In 1999, Schaefer et al (39), reporting results of the Mid European Pediatric Peritoneal Dialysis Study Group, stated that the double-cuff, coiled Tenckhoff catheter had emerged as the standard catheter type in mid Europe. The overall survival rate of the original straight Tenckhoff catheter was 82%, 69%, 60%, and 57% after 1, 2, 3, and 4 years of treatment, respectively. At that time, only 2 out of 15 study centers preferred the Swan Neck catheter. In 2001, guidelines developed by the European Pediatric Peritoneal Dialysis Working Group (40) suggested that a single-cuff catheter may be needed in infants less than 3 kg, but identified the double-cuff coiled catheter as the preferred design in most children (with pediatric size in patients with 3 to 10 kg body weight, and adult catheter in patients > 10 kg). The swan-neck presternal catheter, with the exit site located on the chest wall, is considered particularly useful in patients with specific indications, such as a higher tendency to exit site infections. It also allows safe, long-term PD treatment in very young children with CKD while using diapers (41). In this study of pediatric patients, at the time of presternal catheter insertion the youngest was 2 months old and had a body weight of 3.2 kg.

In children with acute renal failure, the Tenckhoff catheter has been proposed as preferable for acute dialysis, when inserted with a guidewire-based technique. Compared to the trocar-based technique, Tenckhoff catheters inserted percutaneously over a guidewire allow significantly longer periods of dialysis with significantly fewer complications, thus allowing a secure peritoneal access (42).

Catheters for Continuous Flow Peritoneal Dialysis

In the attempt to achieve better depuration with PD, the concept of continuous flow PD (CFPD) has been developed—a treatment characterized by the fact that dialysis fluid flows through the peritoneal cavity at a continuous rate. This can be obtained with 2 single catheters or 1 double-lumen catheter (43,44). Continuous flow PD has the potential of providing increased clearances, up to threefold compared to continuous ambulatory PD (CAPD), thereby avoiding the need for daytime exchanges or reducing the automated PD treatment time (10). Poor mixing of the dialysis fluid and its recirculation pose a major risk of inefficient treatment, with potentially marked variability in terms of clearances and ultrafiltration (UF) rate. Therefore, the 2 catheter tips should be positioned in a way to allow maximum exposure time between the peritoneal surface and the dialysis fluid during the fluid passage from the inflow to the outflow catheter. Double-lumen catheters with intra-abdominal segments of different lengths (one short and the other long, straight or coiled) were originally designed to allow continuous flow (45,46). The evaluation of the efficacy of the new catheters has been limited by several factors, including the fact that in vitro testing of recirculation does not accurately reflect the actual events inside the peritoneal cavity and by the lack of adequate validation of clinical testing protocols (46).

Ash and coworkers have conceived a modified version of the T-fluted catheter, which uses 1 limb of the T-shaped catheter tip for infusion and 1 for drainage (10). Diaz-Buxo (44) described a double-lumen PD catheter with a wide separation between the limbs to minimize streaming and recirculation, and with a novel geometric configuration to maximize internal cross-sectional luminal area with the lowest external diameter. Another double-lumen catheter for CFPD has been designed by Ronco et al. (Figure 5.14) (45,47), with the aim of finding a way to minimize re-circulation. The catheter has a thin-walled proximal inflow diffuser (similar to a flexible shower head) that is positioned at the entry point into the peritoneum. The second lumen, used for drainage, is a long, coiled tube, similar to a conventional coiled catheter. The considerable distance between the 2 lumens and the diffusing effect of the multiple holes in the inflow section may reduce streaming and recirculation.

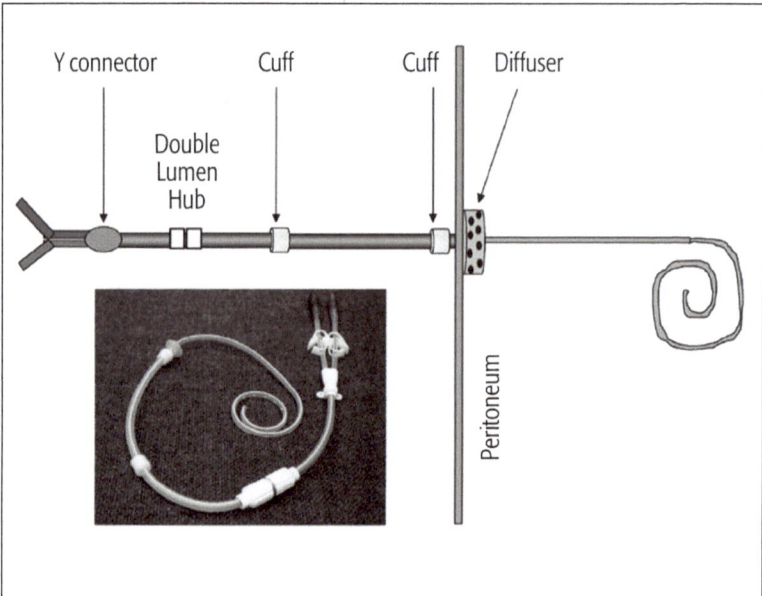

Figure 5.14. Ronco Catheter for CFPD
(Ronco C, Dell'Aquila R, Rodighiero MP, et al. The "Ronco" catheter for continuous flow peritoneal dialysis. *Int J Artif Organs* 2006; 29: 101-12)

REFERENCES

1.   Ash SR. Chronic peritoneal dialysis catheters: Effect of catheter design, materials and location. *Semin Dial* 1990; 3: 39–46.

2.   Ganter G. Uber die Beseitingung giftiger Stoffe aus dem Blute durch Dialyse (On the elimination of toxic substances from the blood by dialysis). *Munch Med Wochenschr* 1923; 70:1478–80.

3.   Grollman A, Turner LB, McLean JA. Intermittent peritoneal lavage in nephrectomized dogs and its application to the human being. *Arch Intern Med* 1951; 87: 376–390.

4.   Maxwell MH, Rockney RE, Kleeman CR, Twiss MR. Peritoneal dialysis. Technique and applications. *JAMA* 1959; 170: 917–24.

5.   Weston RE, Roberts M. Stylet-catheter for peritoneal dialysis. *Lancet* 1965; 285 (7394):1049.

6.   Palmer RA, Quinton WE, Gray JE. Prolonged peritoneal dialysis for chronic renal failure. *Lancet* 1964; 284 (7335): 700–2.

7. Palmer RA. Peritoneal dialysis by indwelling catheter for chronic renal failure 1963–1968. *Can Med Assoc J* 1971; 105: 376–9.

8. Tenckhoff H, Schechter H. A bacteriologically safe peritoneal access device. *Trans Am Soc Artif Intern Organs* 1968; 14: 181–7.

9. Negoi D, Prowant BF, Twardowski ZJ. Current trends in the use of peritoneal dialysis catheters. *Adv Perit Dial* 2006; 22:147–52.

10. Ash SR. Chronic peritoneal dialysis catheters: Challenges and design solutions. *Int J Artif Organs* 2006; 29: 85–94.

11. Strippoli GFM, Tong A, Johnson D, Schena FP, Craig JC. Catheter-related interventions to prevent peritonitis in peritoneal dialysis: A systematic review of randomized, controlled trials. *J Am Soc Nephrol* 2004; 15: 2735–46.

12. Stegmayr BG, Wikdahl AM, Bergstrom M, et al. A randomized clinical trial comparing the function of straight and coiled Tenckhoff catheters for peritoneal dialysis. *Perit Dial Int* 2005; 25:85–88.

13. Twardowski ZJ, Prowant BF, Nichols WK, Nolph KD, Khanna R. Six years experience with swan neck catheter. *Perit Dial Int* 1992; 12:384–9.

14. Sikaneta T, Cheung KM, Abdolell M, et al. The Toronto Western Hospital catheter: one center's experience and review of the literature. *Int J Artif Organs* 2006; 29: 59–63.

15. Twardowski ZJ, Prowant BF, Khanna R, Nichols WK, Nolph KD. Long-term experience with Swan Neck Missouri catheters. *ASAIO Trans* 1990; 36: M491–4.

16. Yerram P, Gill A, Prowant B, Saab G, Misra M, Whaley-Connell A. A 9-year survival analysis of the presternal Missouri swan-neck catheter. *Adv Perit Dial* 2007; 23:90–3.

17. Moncrief JW, Popovich RP. Moncrief-Popovich catheter: Implantation technique and clinical results. *Perit Dial Int* 1994; 14 Suppl 3:S56–8.

18. Dasgupta MK. Moncrief-Popovich catheter and implantation technique: The AV fistula of peritoneal dialysis. *Adv Ren Replace Ther* 2002; 9: 116–24.

19. Brum S, Rodrigues A, Rocha S, et al. Moncrief-Popovich technique is an advantageous method of peritoneal dialysis catheter implantation. *Nephrol Dial Transplant* 2010; 25: 3070–5.

20. Ishizaki M, Suzuki K, Kurosawa K, Shishido Y, Takahashi H. Swan neck Sendai catheter: A modification of the swan neck Tenckhoff catheter. *Perit Dial Int* 1988; 8:221.

21. Twardowski ZJ, Nichols WK, Nolph KD, Khanna R. Swan neck presternal ("bath tub") catheter for peritoneal dialysis. *Adv Perit Dial* 1992; 8:316–24.

22. Twardowski ZJ. Presternal peritoneal catheter. Adv Ren Replace Ther. 2002; 9: 125–32.

23. Cruz C. Clinical experience with a new peritoneal dialysis access device. In: Ota K, Maher J, eds. Current Concepts in Peritoneal Dialysis. *Amsterdam: Elsevier* 1992: 162–9.

24. Crabtree JH. Clinical biodurability of aliphatic polyether based polyurethanes as peritoneal dialysis catheters. *ASAIO J* 2003; 49:290–4.

25. Crabtree JH. Fragmentation of polyurethane peritoneal dialysis catheter during explantation. *Perit Dial int* 2004; 24: 601–2.

26. Ash SR, Sutton JM, Mankus RA, et al. Clinical trials of the T-fluted peritoneal dialysis catheter. *Adv Ren Replace Ther* 2002; 9:133–43.

27. Valli A, Crescimannu U, Midri R. Eighteen months' experience with a new (Valli) catheter for peritoneal dialysis. *Perit Dial Bull* 1983; 3:107–9.

28. Dell'Aquila R, Chiaramonte S, Rodighiero MO, et al. The Vicenza "Short" peritoneal catheter: A twenty-year experience. *Int J Artif Organs* 2006; 29: 123–127.

29. Twardowski ZJ. Malposition and poor drainage of peritoneal catheters. *Semin Dial* 1990; 3: 57.

30. Vogt K, Binswanger U, Buchman P. Catheter-related complications during CAPD: A retrospective study on sixty-two double-cuff Tenckhoff catheters. *Am J Kidney Dis* 1987; 10:47–51.

31. Di Paolo N, Petrini G, Garosi G, Buoncristiani U, Berardi S, Monaci G. A new self-locating peritoneal catheter. *Perit Dial Int* 1996; 16:623–7.

32. Di Paolo N, Capotondo L, Brardi S, Nicolai G. The self-locating peritoneal catheter: Fifteen years of experience. *Perit Dial Int* 2010; 30: 504–5.

33. Di Paolo N, Capotondo L, Sansoni E, et al. The self-locating catheter: clinical experience and follow-up. *Perit Dial Int* 2004; 24: 359–64.

34. Vigneux A, Hardy BE, Balfe JW. Chronic peritoneal catheter in children -one or two dacron cuffs? (Letter) *Perit Dial Bull* 1981; 1: 151.

35. Watson AR, Vigneux A, Hardy BE, Balfe JW. Six years' experience with CAPD catheters in children. *Perit Dial Bull* 1985; 5: 119–122.

36. Lewis MA, Smith T, Postlethwaite RJ, Webb NJ. A comparison of double-cuffed with single-cuffed Tenckhoff catheters in the prevention of infection in pediatric patients. *Adv Perit Dial* 1997; 13:274–6.

37. Rinaldi S, Sera F, Verrina E, et al. The Italian registry of pediatric chronic peritoneal dialysis: A ten-year experience with chronic peritoneal dialysis catheters. *Perit Dial Int* 1998; 18:71–4.

38. Alexander SR, Donaldson LA, Sullivan EK. CAPD/ CCPD for children in North America: the NAPRTCS experience. In: Fine RN, Alexander SR, Warady BA, eds. CAPD/CCPD in Children. *Boston: Kluwer Academic Publishers* 1998; 1–16.

39. Schaefer F, Klaus G, Muller, Wiefel DE, Mehls O. Current practice of peritoneal dialysis in children: Results of a longitudinal survey. Mid European Pediatric Peritoneal Dialysis Study Group (MEPPS). *Perit Dial Int* 1999; 19(Suppl 2):S445–9.

40. Watson AR, Gartland C. European Paediatric Peritoneal Dialysis Working Group. Guidelines by an ad hoc European committee for elective chronic peritoneal dialysis in pediatric patients. *Perit Dial Int* 2001; 21:240–4.

41. Warchol S, Roszkowska–Blaim M, Latoszynska J, Jarmolinski T, Zachwieja J. Experience using presternal catheter for peritoneal dialysis in Poland: A multicenter pediatric survey. *Perit Dial Int* 2003; 23:242–248

42. Lewis MA, Nycyk JA. Practical peritoneal dialysis--the Tenckhoff catheter in acute renal failure. Pediatr Nephrol. 1992; 6: 470–5.

43. Cruz C, Melendez A, Gotch FA, Folden T, Crawford T, Diaz—Buxo JA. Single-pass continuous flow peritoneal dialysis using two catheters. *Semin Dial* 2001; 14:391–4.

44. Diaz-Buxo JA. Streaming, mixing, and recirculation: Role of the peritoneal access in continuous flow peritoneal dialysis (clinical considerations). *Adv Perit Dial* 2002; 18: 87–90.

45. Ronco C, Dell'Aquila R, Bonello M, et al. Continuous flow peritoneal dialysis: A new double lumen catheter. *Int J Artif Organs* 2003; 26: 984–90.

46. Diaz-Buxo JA. Access and continuous flow peritoneal dialysis. *Perit Dial Int* 2005; 25 (Suppl. 3): S102–4.

47. Ronco C, Dell'Aquila R, Rodighiero MP, et al. The "Ronco" catheter for continuous flow peritoneal dialysis. *Int J Artif Organs* 2006; 29: 101–12.

POSTSURGICAL CARE OF A PERITONEAL DIALYSIS CATHETER

Please refer to the "Appendix of Peritoneal Dialysis Products Cited in this Volume" for a list of companies that are holding copyrights or selling specific products cited in this chapter.

J. BARDSLEY, S. McMICHAEL

CONNECTING A BAXTER TRANSFER SET TO A PERITONEAL DIALYSIS CATHETER

The transfer set provides a fluid pathway between the PD catheter and the dialysate tubing. If the transfer set was not attached by the surgeon, a PD nurse will connect a transfer set to the patient's catheter prior to initiating PD. For ease of explanation, this section discusses the Baxter system for delivery. There are other delivery systems available, and the choice of system will be determined by the facility or physician. The Fresenius system is described in this chapter's section on flushing a catheter.

The procedure for connecting a transfer set to the patient's catheter is performed using a strict, sterile technique. The procedure is done in an outpatient dialysis clinic, by a registered nurse. It takes about 10 minutes to complete. The transfer set should be replaced every 6 months or sooner if the device is compromised—for instance, a hole or break develops in the catheter.

NOTE: This procedure requires strict sterile technique.

Table 6.1. Supplies for Connecting Transfer Set to PD Catheter (Figure 6.1)

Number In Set	Supplies
2	sterile barriers
2	pair of sterile gloves
1	MiniCap
1	transfer set
1	beta clamp
2 or more	face masks
1	bottle of Alcavis 50
1	roll of surgical tape
3	packages of 4 × 4 inch gauze

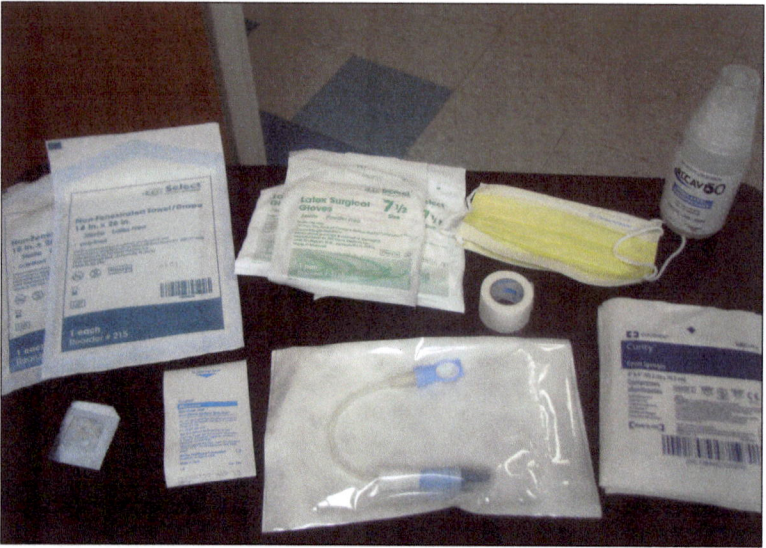

Figure 6.1. Unopened Sterile Supplies for Connecting Transfer Set to PD Catheter

Procedure

1. Remove the patient's clothing.

2. Place the supplies on a clean dry surface (Figure 6.1).

3. Don face masks to prevent infection. Everyone in the room must wear a mask.

4. Wash hands for 1 minute.

5. Open the first sterile barrier and place it on a table.

6. Open the following packages and place the contents on the sterile barrier, without touching the sterile items: MiniCap, transfer set, 4 × 4 inch gauze.

7. Open the second sterile barrier and place it under the PD catheter up to the exit site, in order to create a sterile field. (If this is an exchange procedure rather than an initial connection, place the PD catheter and the old transfer set on top of the sterile barrier.)

8. Use the beta clamp to occlude the PD catheter near the exit site.

9. Pour Alcavis 50 over two 4 × 4 inch gauze pads.

10. Don sterile gloves.

11. Close the twist clamp on the new transfer set.

12. Remove the protective cover from the blue end of the transfer set and discard.

13. Place the MiniCap on the blue end of the new transfer set.

14. Place an Alcavis-soaked 4 × 4 inch gauze around the catheter adapter. Cleanse the adapter for one minute to sterilize the inside of the catheter adapter. Leave the gauze in place around the adapter. (Figure 6.2)

15. Remove and discard contaminated gloves; don new sterile gloves.

16. To prevent contamination of sterile gloves by the PD catheter, hold the PD catheter with a dry, sterile 4 × 4 inch gauze. With the other hand, remove the Alcavis-soaked 4 × 4 inch gauze from the catheter adapter.

17. Place a dry, sterile 4 × 4 inch gauze under the catheter.

18. While still holding the PD catheter with a dry, sterile 4 × 4 inch gauze, securely attach the new transfer set to the PD catheter. The purpose of the gauze is to prevent contamination of the sterile gloves and to aid in making a secure attachment to the catheter. (Figure 6.3)

19. Remove the beta clamp from the PD catheter.

20. Avoid placing any tension on the catheter and secure it to the abdomen with surgical tape so that the catheter is not pulling at the exit site.

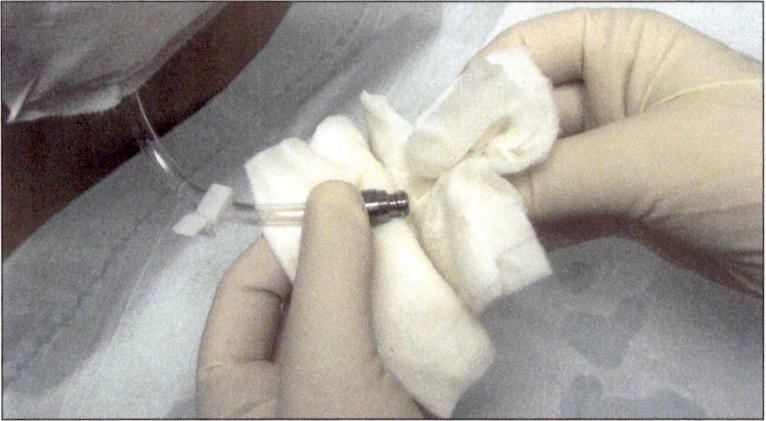

Figure 6.2. Cleanse PD Adapter
Using sterile technique, cleanse the adaptor at the end of the PD catheter for one minute with Alcavis.

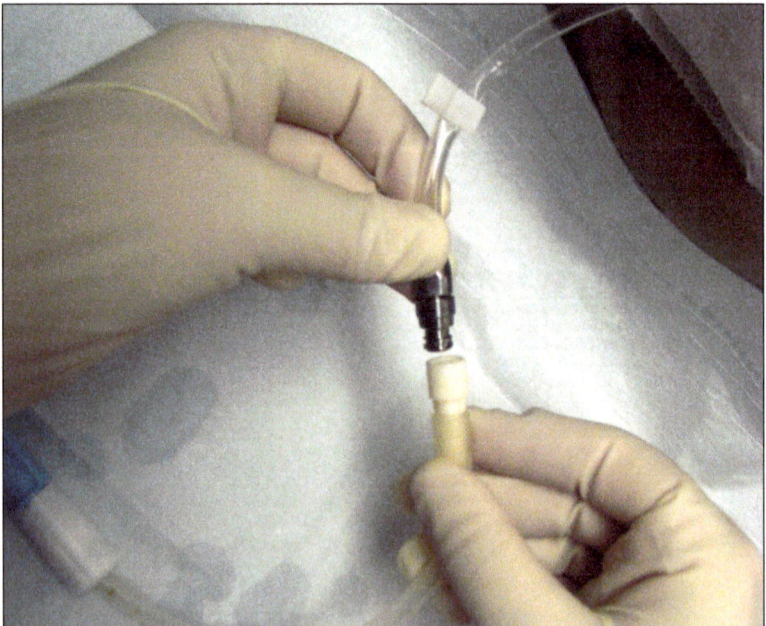

Figure 6.3. Attach New Transfer Set to PD Catheter
Donning sterile gloves and a face mask, attach the new transfer set securely to the PD catheter. The gauze described in Step 18 is omitted from this figure in the interest of clearly depicting the instrumentation.

FIRST POSTOPERATIVE CATHETER DRESSING CHANGE

In surgery, the operative site is dressed under sterile conditions immediately after placement of the PD catheter. The PD nurse will remove the non-occlusive dressing when the patient is seen for the first catheter flush, 3 to 5 days after PD catheter placement.

Table 6.2. Supplies for First Postoperative Catheter Dressing Change (Figure 6.4)

Number In Set	Supplies
1	bottle of ExSept Plus
2 or more	face masks
1	pair of non-sterile gloves
1	pair of sterile gloves
1	package of sterile 4 × 4 inch gauze
1	sterile barrier
1	package of sterile 2 × 2 inch gauze (optional)
1	Tegaderm dressing (optional)
1	Biopatch (optional)

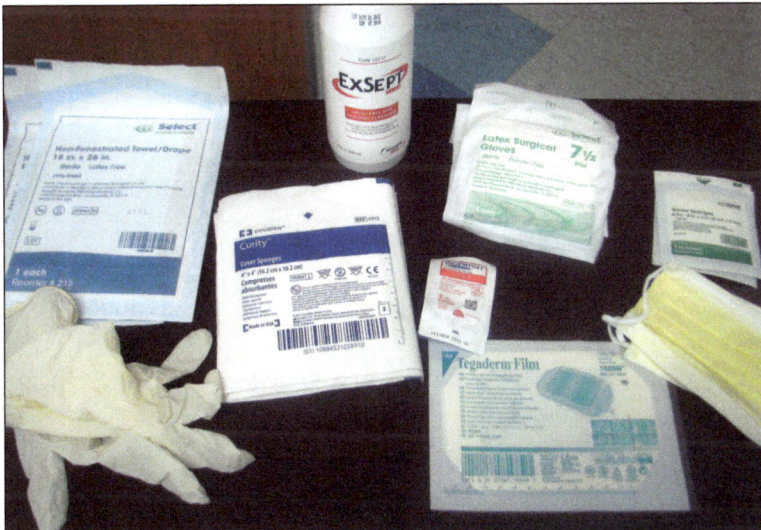

Figure 6.4. Unopened Sterile Supplies for First Postoperative Dressing Change

Procedure

■ 1. Don face masks to prevent infection. Everyone in the room must wear a mask.

■ 2. Wash hands for 1 minute.

■ 3. Open a sterile barrier and place it under the PD catheter up to the exit site.

■ 4. Don non-sterile gloves, remove the old dressing, and discard it.

■ 5. Remove non-sterile gloves and wash hands.

■ 6. Open a second sterile barrier and place it on a table.

■ 7. Open 4 packages of 4 × 4 inch gauze and place them on the sterile barrier.

■ 8. Soak 1 package of 4 × 4 inch gauze with ExSept.

■ 9. Open the Biopatch and Tegaderm packages.

■ 10. Don sterile gloves.

■ 11. Thoroughly cleanse the skin around the catheter using 4 × 4 inch gauze soaked with ExSept. Work from the exit site and suture line outward using a separate gauze for each site. Do not allow solution to enter the sinus tract. (Figure 6.5)

■ 12. Allow the skin to dry (a dry, sterile 4 × 4 inch gauze may be used to dry the area).

■ 13. Apply the Biopatch around the exit site (Figure 6.6) then cover it with either a 2 × 2 inch or 4 × 4 inch gauze, followed by a Tegaderm dressing (Figure 6.7).

■ 14. Avoid placing any tension on the catheter and secure it to the abdomen with surgical tape so that the catheter is not pulling at the exit site (Figure 6.8).

The dressing should remain in place for 5 to 7 days. If the dressing becomes saturated, patients may reinforce the dressing and call a PD nurse.

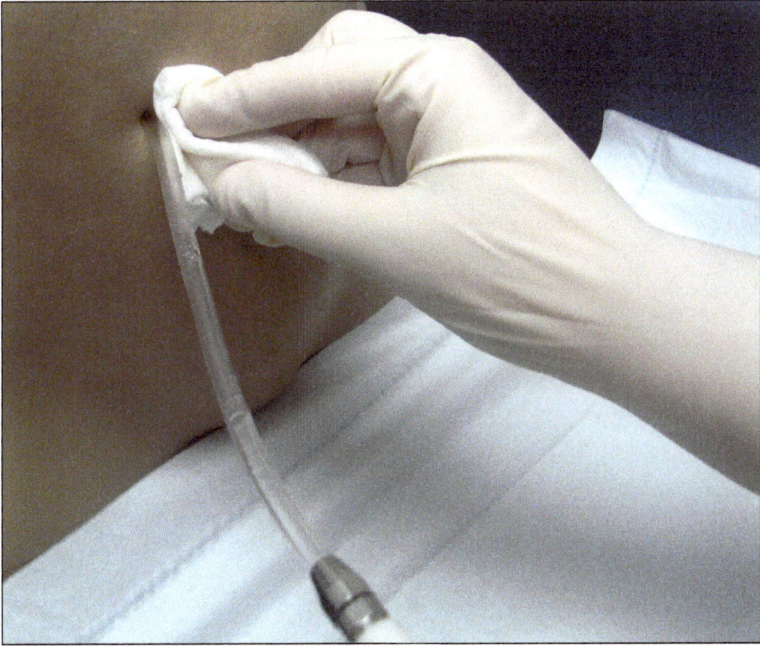

Figure 6.5. Cleanse Skin Surrounding Catheter
Cleanse the skin surrounding the catheter using a 4 × 4 inch gauze soaked with ExSept.

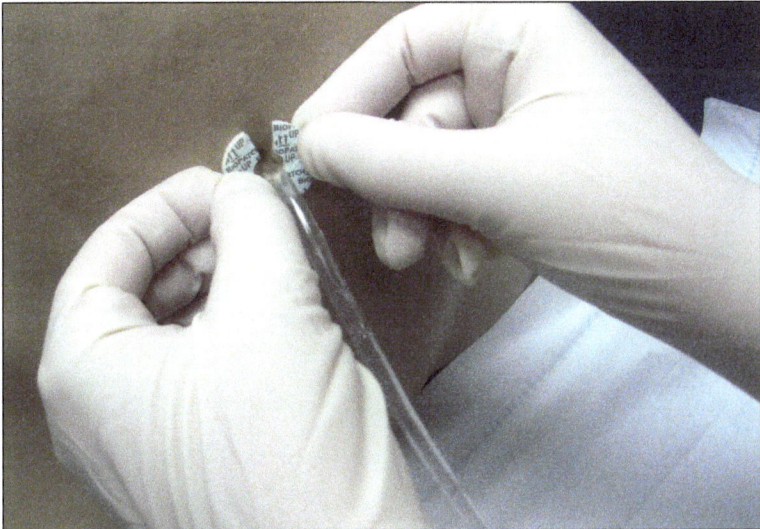

Figure 6.6. Biopatch Placed around Catheter at Skin Exit Site

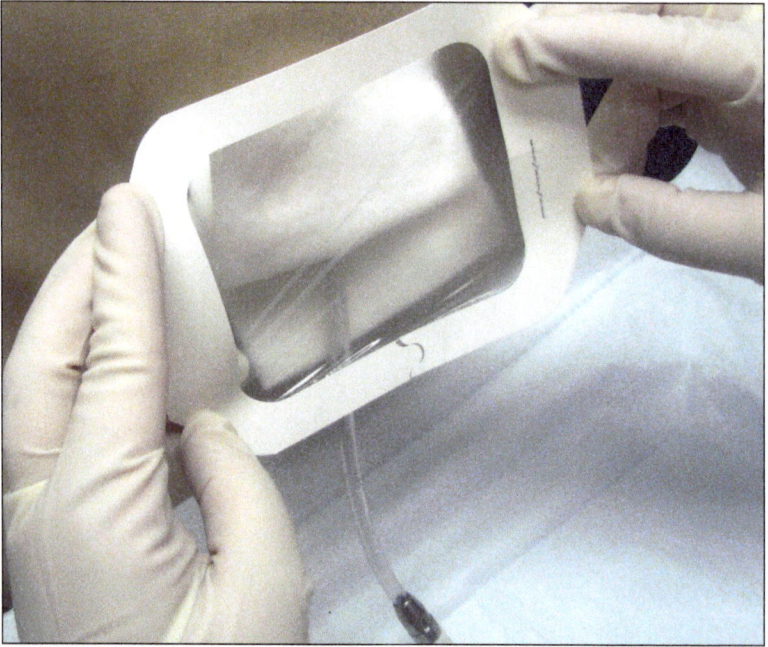

Figure 6.7. Tegaderm Dressing Applied over Gauze and Part of Catheter

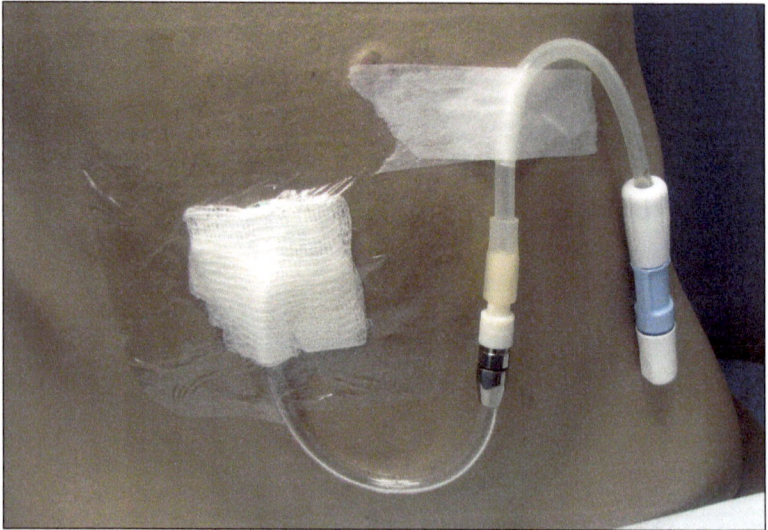

Figure 6.8. Dressing Change Complete
Tension and pulling on the catheter at the exit site is avoided by positioning and taping the transfer set to the abdomen, leaving slack in the tubing.

THE BAXTER SYSTEM FOR FLUSHING A CATHETER

Patients are seen by a PD nurse 3 to 5 days after placement of the catheter, for an initial flush, usually done in conjunction with the first sterile dressing change. Flushing the catheter ensures catheter patency and proper placement. This procedure should be performed weekly (or bi-weekly) until PD training begins. Flushing is to be performed in a clinic room, with the doors closed.

Table 6.3. Supplies for Flushing PD Catheter (Figure 6.9)

Number In Set	Supplies
1	Ultrabag
2	MiniCaps
2	clamps
1	syringe (3 cc or 10 cc)
1	bottle of Alcavis 50
1	roll of surgical tape
1	bottle of hand sanitizer
1	vial of heparin (1000 units/liter)
1	IV pole
1	spring scale
2 or more	face masks

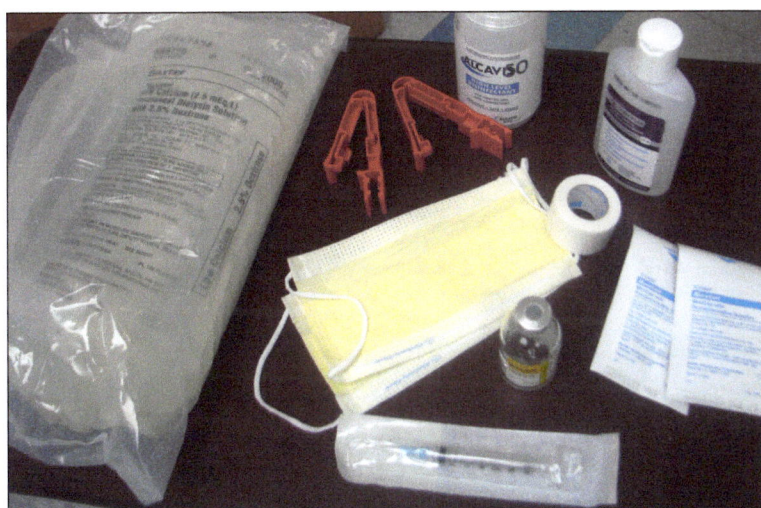

Figure 6.9. Unopened Supplies for Flushing PD Catheter

Procedure

■ 1. Gather supplies. Check the UltraBag for the correct dextrose concentration and current expiration date. Warm the UltraBag in its overwrap.

■ 2. Don face mask and wash hands for 1 minute.

■ 3. Remove the warmed UltraBag from its overwrap.

■ 4. Apply enough Alcavis solution to sterilize the medication port on the UltraBag and the top of the heparin vial (Figures 6.10 and 6.11).

■ 5. Wait one minute.

■ 6. Add heparin (1000 units per liter) to the UltraBag, using sterile technique (Figure 6.12).

■ 7. Separate and uncoil the tubing.

■ 8. Hang the UltraBag on the spring scale attached to the IV pole (Figure 6.13).

■ 9. Lay the drain bag on floor, with the shiny side up.

■ 10. Break the blue frangible (Figure 6.14) and connect the Y connector set to the patient's transfer set (Figure 6.15).

■ 11. Clamp the tubing to the UltraBag and break the green frangible.

■ 12. Open the twist clamp on the transfer set to drain any effluent that may be present. There will most likely be no effluent, as the abdominal cavity is typically dry at this stage.

■ 13. Close the twist clamp on the transfer set.

■ 14. To flush the air from the tubing, remove the clamp from the tubing to the UltraBag for 5 seconds and place it on the tubing to the drain bag.

■ 15. Open the twist clamp on the transfer set (Figure 6.16).

■ 16. Allow 500 cc of heparinized dialysate to instill.

17. After 500 cc is instilled, remove the clamp from the tubing to the drain bag and place it on the tubing to the UltraBag.

18. Allow the entire 500 cc of dialysate to drain into the drain bag.

19. Repeat Steps 16 through 18, for a total of 1500 cc of dialysate instilled and drained.

20. Close the twist clamp on the transfer set.

21. Place one clamp on the tubing to the UltraBag and one clamp on the tubing to the drain bag.

22. Don new masks and wash hands.

23. Open the MiniCap package, keeping it sterile.

24. Disconnect the Y connector from the patient's transfer set (Figure 6.17).

25. Apply a new sterile MiniCap to the transfer set (Figure 6.18).

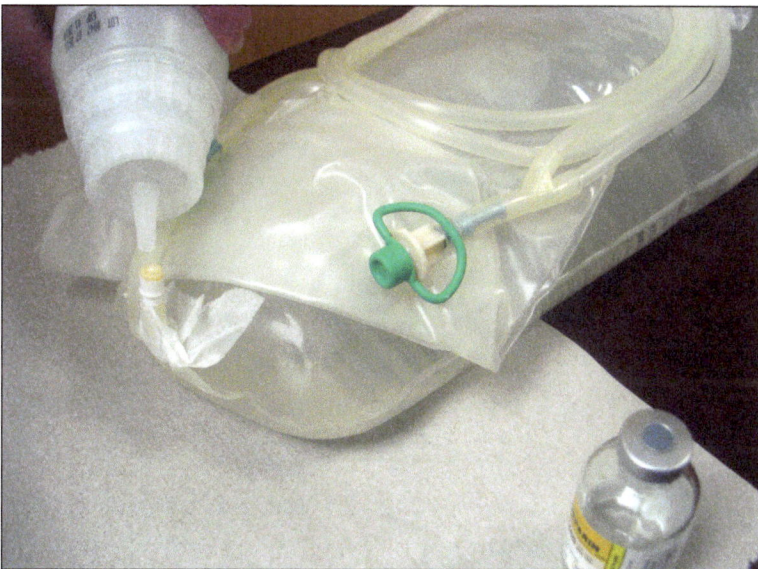

Figure 6.10. Sterilize UltraBag Port with Alcavis

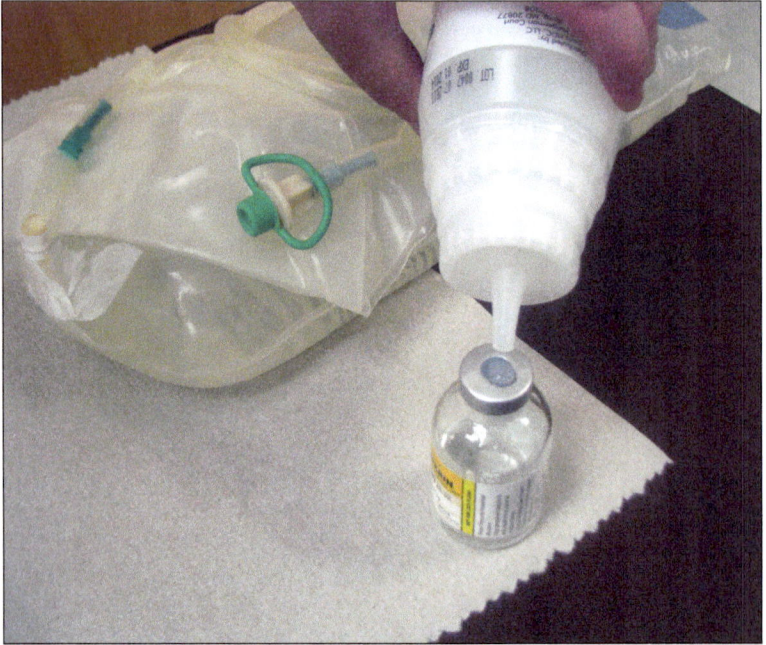

Figure 6.11. Sterilize Heparin Vial with Alcavis

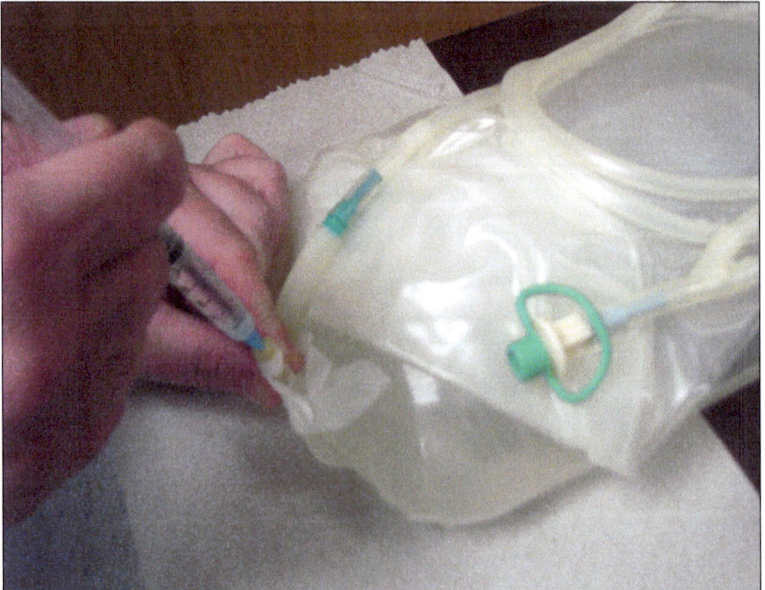

Figure 6.12. Inject Heparin (1000 units/liter) into Medication Port on Dialysate Bag

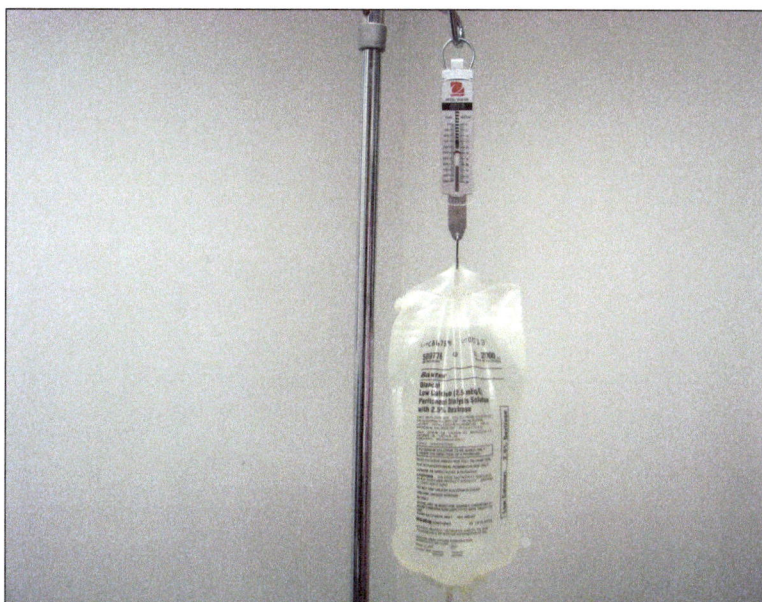

Figure 6.13. Hang Heparinized Dialysate Bag on Spring Scale

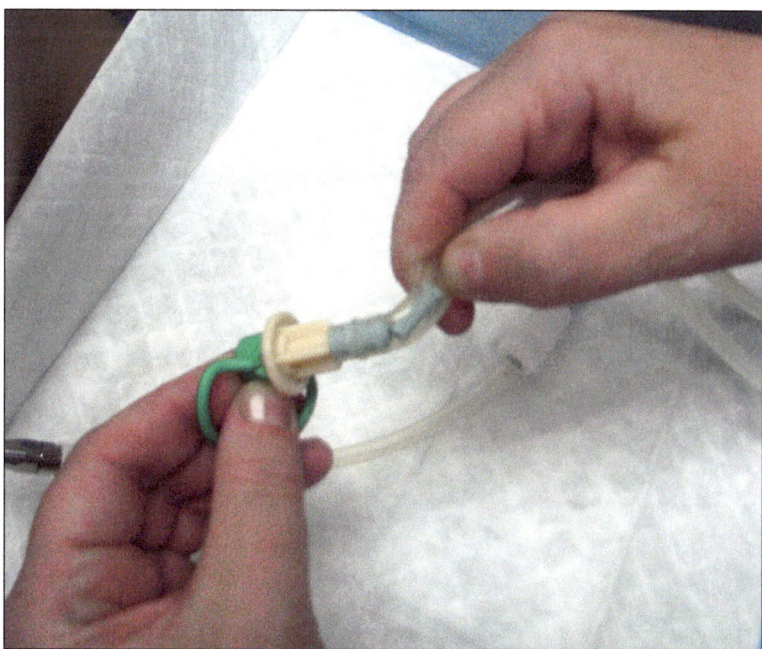

Figure 6.14. Break Blue Frangible at Y Connector

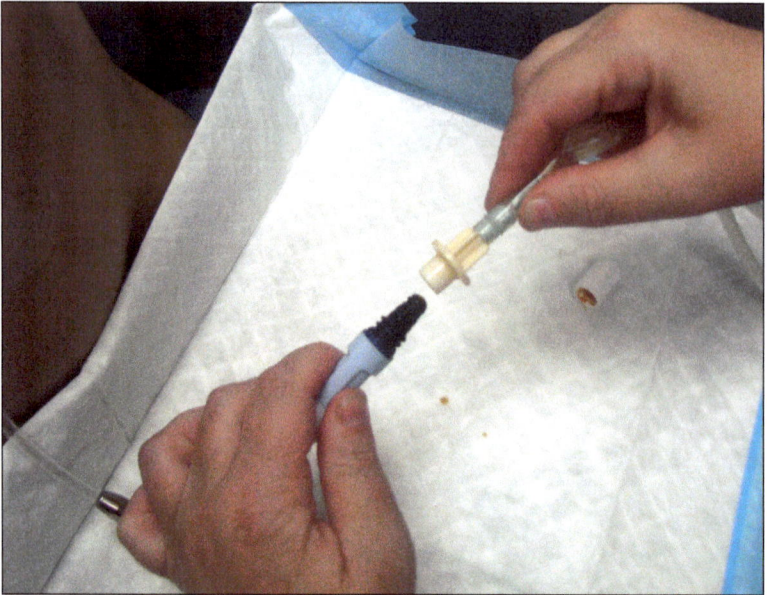

Figure 6.15. Connect Y Connector to Patient's Transfer Set (Sterile Connection)

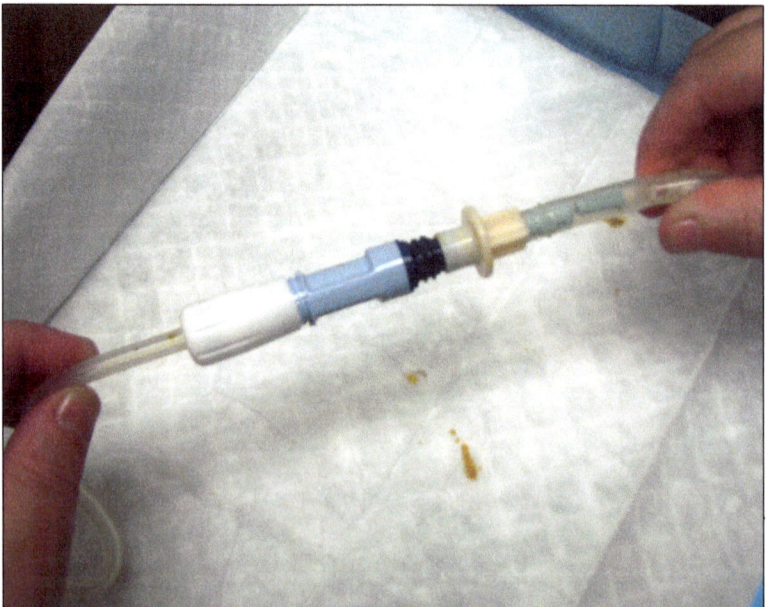

Figure 6.16. Open Twist Clamp on Patient's Transfer Set and Flush Catheter Following Steps 16 through 20

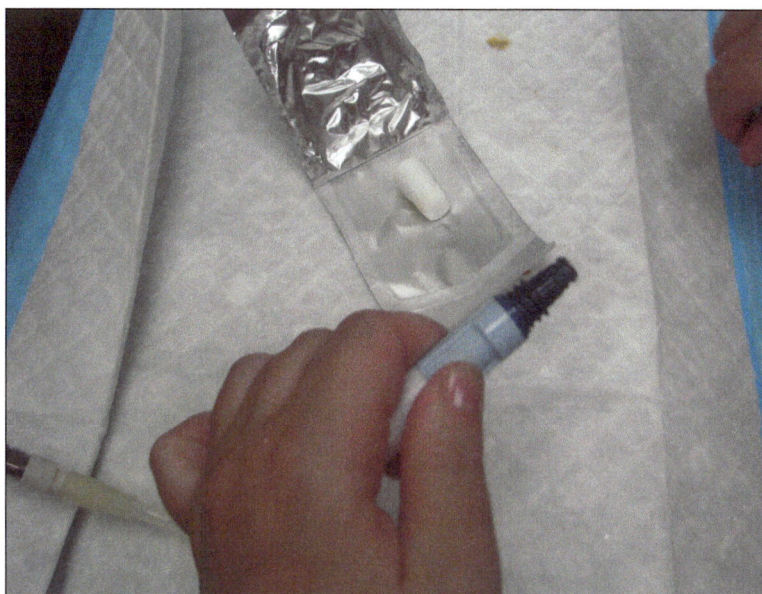

Figure 6.17. After Flushing: Open New Sterile MiniCap; Disconnect Y Connector from Patient's Transfer Set

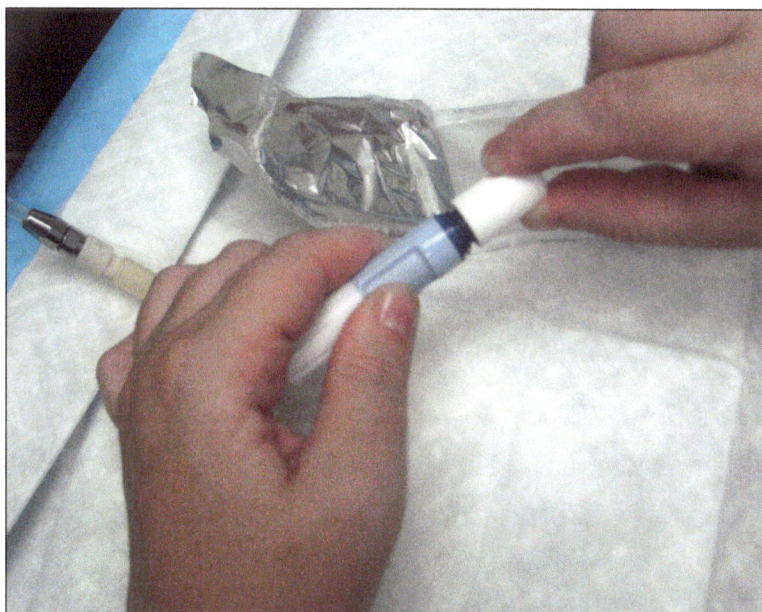

Figure 6.18. Apply New Sterile MiniCap to Transfer Set

THE FRESENIUS STAY-SAFE SYSTEM FOR FLUSHING A CATHETER

The Stay-Safe system uses a disc, which is a central control dial that prompts the care provider through the treatment steps. No clamps are required with this system—the dial is used to advance from one step to the next.

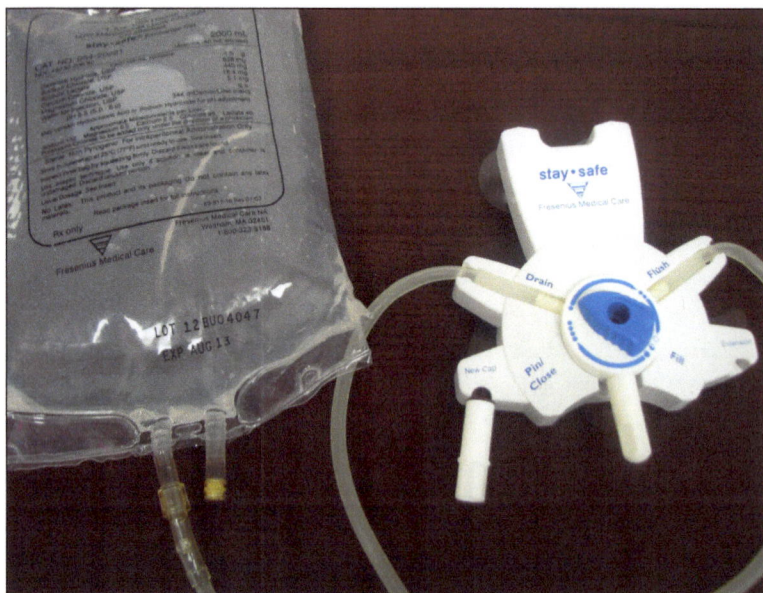

Figure 6.19. Fresenius Stay-Safe System with Central Control-dial Disc

Procedure

1. Gather supplies. Check the solution bag for the correct dextrose concentration and current expiration date. Warm the solution bag in its overwrap.

2. Don face mask and wash hands for 1 minute.

3. Remove the warmed solution bag from its overwrap.

4. Apply enough Alcavis solution to sterilize the medication port on the solution bag and the top of the heparin vial.

5. Wait one minute.

6. Add heparin (1000 units per liter) to the solution bag, using sterile technique.

7. Separate and uncoil the tubing.

8. Hang the solution bag on the spring scale attached to the IV pole.

9. Lay the drain bag on floor, with the shiny side up.

10. Place the Stay-Safe disc in the organizer, as directed.

11. Break the frangible in the line to the hanging solution bag.

12. Place a new cap in the "New Cap" notch in the organizer.

13. Connect the patient's catheter to the Stay-Safe system by first inserting the cap that is attached to the end of the catheter extension set into the "Extension" notch of the organizer.

14. Remove the protective cap from the Stay-Safe disc.

15. Unscrew the extension set from its cap. The cap will remain in the "Extension" notch of the organizer.

16. Immediately connect the catheter extension set to the connector on the bottom of the Stay-Safe disc.

17. Open the clamp on the patient's catheter extension set.

18. To drain, turn the dial to the position labeled "Drain."

19. To flush the lines, turn the dial to the position labeled "Flush."

20. To fill, turn the dial to the position labeled "Fill." Stop at 500 ml.

21. Turn the dial back to "Drain" to drain out that 500 ml.

22. Repeat Steps 20 and 21 twice more, for a total of 3 fill-and-drain sessions of 500 ml, using a total of 1500 ml of solution.

■ 23. The dial must be turned to the "Pin/Close" position at the completion of the flushes so that the closure pin from the disc will be inserted into the patient's extension set.

■ 24. Close the clamp on the patient's extension set and unscrew the protective cover from the new Stay-Safe cap.

■ 25. Unscrew the extension set from the disc.

■ 26. Immediately attach the extension set to the new Stay-Safe cap and remove it from the organizer.

DAILY EXIT SITE CARE

Approximately one week after the first sterile dressing change, a PD nurse will educate the patient on non-sterile daily exit site care to prevent infection. To promote uniform healing of the exit site and to prevent tissue overgrowth, it is recommended that the catheter be taped to the abdomen in the 3-6-9-12 positions, rotating the position each time the dressing is changed.

Table 6.4. Supplies for Daily Exit Site Care (Figure 6.19)

Number In Set	Supplies
1	bottle of ExSept Plus
1	package of sterile 4 × 4 inch gauze
3	packages of sterile 2 × 2 inch gauze
1	bottle of hand sanitizer
1	tube of gentamicin 0.1% cream
1	roll of surgical tape

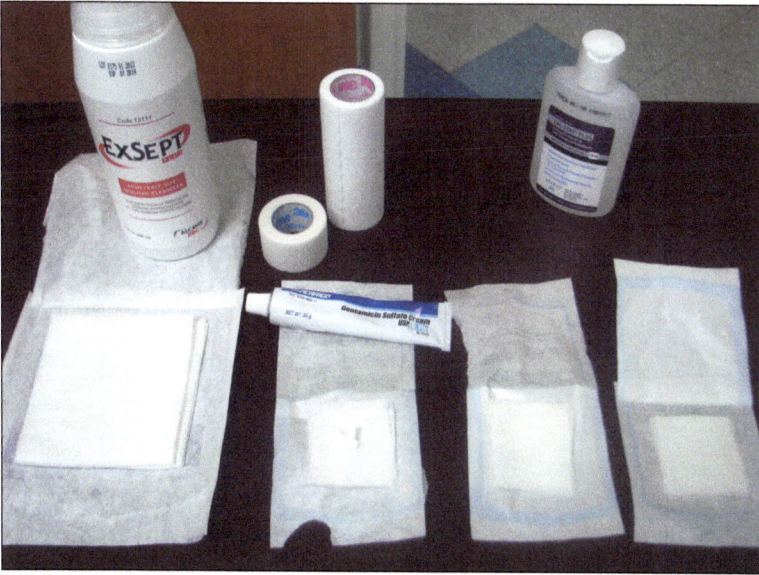

Figure 6.20. Daily Care Supplies
Daily care supplies include aseptic solution, 4 × 4 inch and 2 × 2 inch sterile gauze, hand sanitizer, 0.1% gentamicin cream, and surgical tape.

Procedure

1. Gather supplies.

2. Wash hands for 1 minute.

3. Remove old dressing and discard.

4. Apply hand sanitizer.

5. Open the 4 × 4 inch and the 2 × 2 inch gauze packages and soak one 4 × 4 gauze with ExSept.

6. Apply a small amount of gentamicin 0.1 % cream to the center of a 2 × 2 inch gauze.

7. Beginning at the exit site, wipe the area with an ExSept-soaked 4 × 4 inch gauze, in a circular motion, moving outward.

8. Allow to dry.

■ 9.   Apply gentamicin cream around the exit site with a 2 × 2 inch gauze
       (Figure 6.21). Discard the gauze.

■ 10. Place a 2 × 2 inch gauze under the catheter and place a 2 × 2 inch gauze
       over the exit site.

■ 11. With a small piece of tape, attach the catheter to the abdomen, leaving
       slack in the tubing.

■ 12. Use tape to secure the gauze.

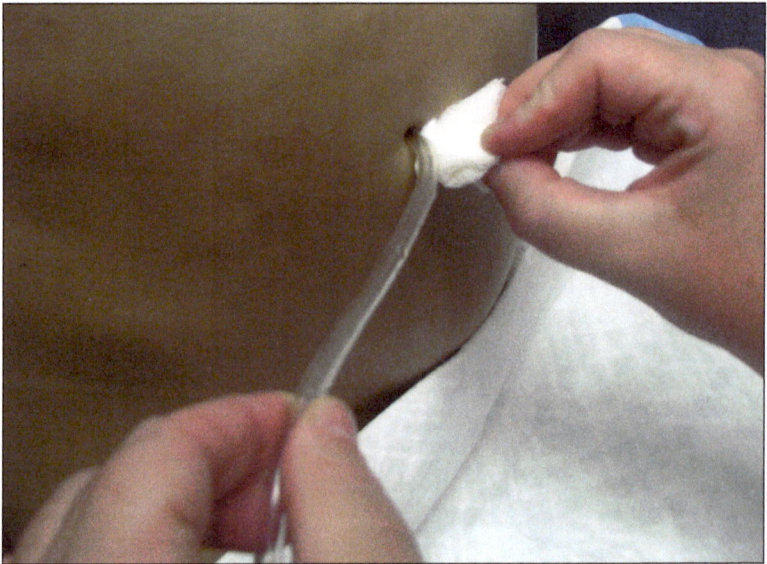

Figure 6.21 Cleanse Skin at Exit Site and Apply Gentamicin Cream
With ExSept-soaked gauze, cleanse the skin around the exit site in a circular motion,
moving outward. Use a second ExSept-soaked gauze to cleanse the tube, working from
the exit site outward. A small amount of 0.1% gentamicin cream is then applied at the
exit site.

POSTSURGICAL INSTRUCTIONS FOR PATIENTS

The following are instructions you may want to pass on to new PD patients.

Your catheter is your lifeline. It is important that you care for it and protect it.

- You should always have a dressing over the catheter.
- A PD nurse will change your dressing for you so you will need to make an appointment for this approximately one week after surgery.
- Keep the dressing dry and intact until you see your PD nurse.
- To keep the dressing dry, bathe yourself using a washcloth and mild soap.
- Avoid the shower and tub.
- You may be sore, so keep activity light.
- Take pain medication, stool softeners, and laxatives as needed.

Report any of the following to your home training clinic:

- Severe Cough
- Constipation/straining to have a bowel movement
- If your dressing is wet, bloody (fresh), or loose

Sample Letter to a New PD Patient

Hello Mr./Ms. Smith,

This information packet is being sent to welcome you to the Home Dialysis Program. You will find a list of items that you may want to obtain prior to starting your peritoneal dialysis training. You will find important information about your catheter as well as when and how you can page or phone a peritoneal dialysis nurse. We look forward to working with you.

Sincerely,

The Home Modality Team

A CLINICAL NEPHROLOGY REVIEW

R. SAXENA

BACKGROUND

The population of the United States is experiencing an exponential growth of ESRD requiring RRT. There were over 571,414 patients with ESRD in 2009, consuming 8.1 % of the Medicare budget and $42.5 billion in total costs (1). With an annual growth of 4%, the ESRD population is projected to grow to more than 775,000 patients on dialysis in 2020 (1). Currently there are 3 RRT options, renal transplant, HD and PD. While renal transplant remains the RRT of choice, the proportion of patients with ESRD receiving renal transplant has not changed in the past decade (1). With increasing number of patients with ESRD requiring dialysis, one would expect a proportionate growth of the 2 dialysis modalities. On the contrary however, while utilization of HD has progressively increased, there has been a steady decline the PD usage, with about 6.9 % of total USA patients on dialysis receiving PD in 2009 (1) (Figures 7.1 and 7.2). In contrast, PD is employed much more frequently elsewhere in the world (Figure 7.3) and is the primary mode of dialysis therapy in Mexico (1).

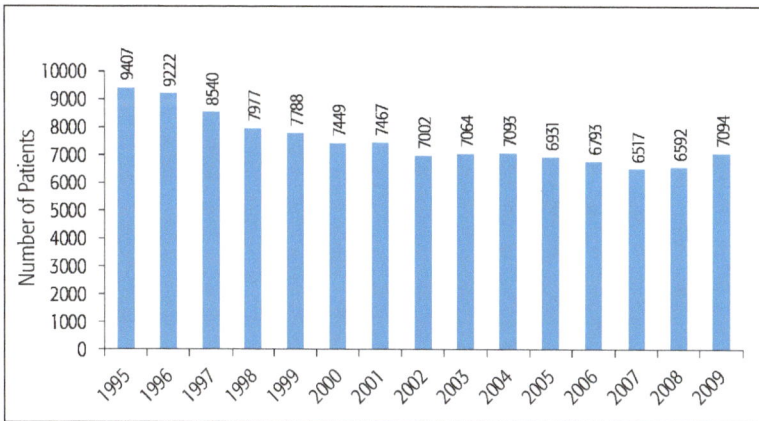

Figure 7.1. Number of Incident PD Patients 1995–2009
(United States Renal Data System, *Annual Data Report* 2011, Bethesda, MD)

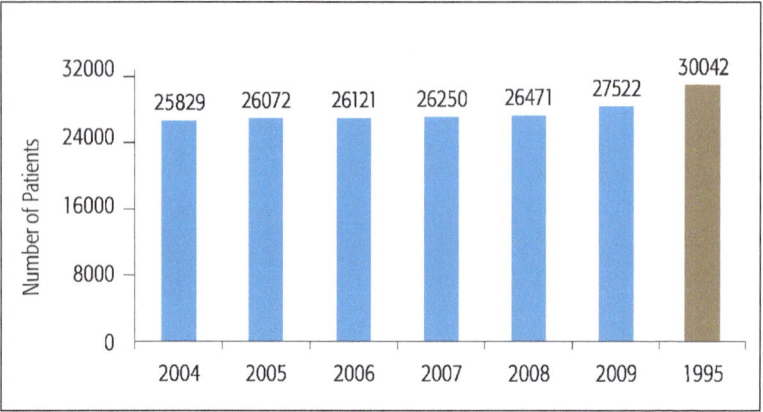

Figure 7.2. Number of Prevalent PD Patients 1995–2009
(United States Renal Data System, *Annual Data Report* 2011, Bethesda.MD)

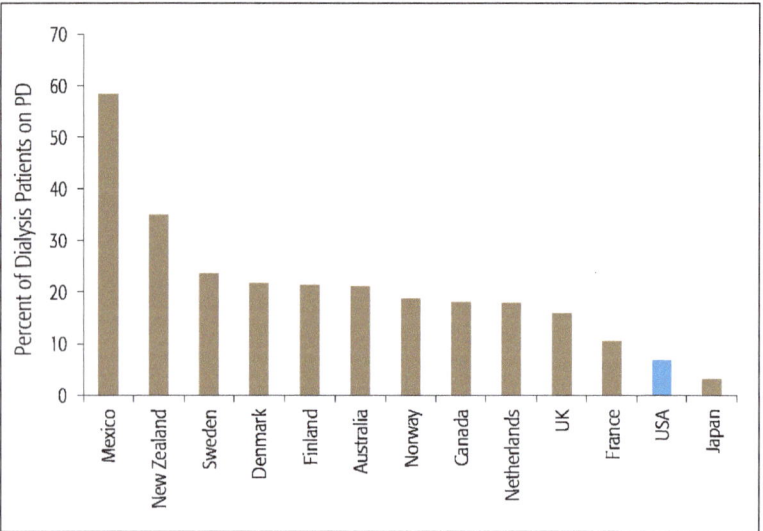

Figure 7.3. Percent of ESRD Patients on PD in Various Countries
(United States Renal Data System, *Annual Data Report* 2011, Bethesda.MD)

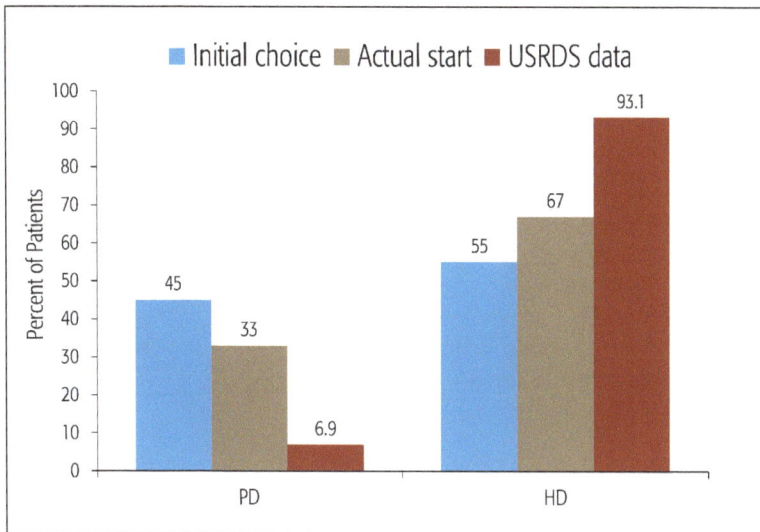

Figure 7.4. Impact of Patient Education on Modality Selection
National pre-ESRD education initiative, preliminary results. Abbreviation: USRDS, United States Renal Data System.

The reasons for minimal utilization of PD in the USA are influenced by psychosocial and economic factors, physician bias, and inadequate pre-ESRD education to the patient (2). Firstly, exposure to PD during nephrology fellowship is paltry (3). A practicing nephrologist with inadequate PD training will be reluctant to offer this therapy to the patients (4). Lack of pre-ESRD education is a key factor that has contributed to a regression of the population of patients on PD in the USA. The USRDS Dialysis Morbidity and Mortality Wave 2 study drew attention to the lack of pre-ESRD education among patients with CKD. It was noted that among new patients with onset of ESRD who are initiating HD, only 25% of the patients reported PD being discussed with them before they started treatment for kidney failure (2). Since then, rates of discussion of PD among patients with CKD have increased as suggested by the recent Comprehensive Dialysis Study, comprising a cohort of incident patients beginning dialysis in the 2005–2007 period (4). In this study, it was observed that 61% of the patients reported that PD had been discussed with them before the start of dialysis. However, only 11% of the patients informed about PD as an option actually chose this modality. This parallels the decline in PD utilization countrywide in the corresponding period. The low rate of PD acceptance among informed patients in the study is likely a result of quality and quantity of information presented to the patients as a part of their pre-ESRD education. The importance of quality patient education is underscored by the results of the National Pre-ESRD Education Initiative where 45% of the patients who received pre-ESRD education opted for PD and 33% actually started PD (5). Similarly, in a report from Hong Kong, 50% patients who were offered PD were reluctant to start PD initially but agreed after predialysis counseling (6). Another report from United Kingdom showed that close to 50% patients who receive explanations for PD and HD through predialysis counseling would choose PD (7). (Figure 7.4)

Thus, in order to enhance utilization of PD in the USA, greater effort should be made to improve PD education during medical fellowship training, and to present clear and accurate pre-ESRD education to each patient. A multidisciplinary pre-ESRD education program that includes nephrologists, nurses, dieticians, and social workers can considerably enhance the use of PD.

INTRODUCTION

Peritoneal dialysis is achieved by instilling dialysis solution into the peritoneal cavity using a percutaneous abdominal catheter. The natural membrane lining the peritoneal cavity acts as a dialysis membrane. Interestingly, when the abdominal cavity is filled with dialysis solution via an abdominal catheter, ancient phylogenic conditions are recreated. Coelomic cavity is the most primitive excretory organ. Even in certain species of fish, the peritoneal cavity is full of liquid and communicates with the external environment through a small passage, analogous to a peritoneal catheter in patients on PD (8).

THE PERITONEAL CAVITY

The peritoneal cavity is the largest serosal cavity in the body, lined by a thin (40μm) layer of peritoneum, consisting of a mesothelium monolayer and underlying connective tissue interstitium. It covers the inner surface of the abdominal wall (parietal peritoneum, 10–15%) and the majority of visceral organs (visceral peritoneum 85–90%) and has a surface area of 1–2 m2. The visceral peritoneum gets its vascular supply from mesenteric arteries and the portal vein, whereas arteries and veins of the abdominal wall supply the parietal peritoneum. The peritoneal blood flow is about 60–70 ml/min. Lymphatic drainage from the peritoneal cavity is through interstitial lymphatics and sub-diaphragmatic lymph stomata (9,10). (Figure 7.5)

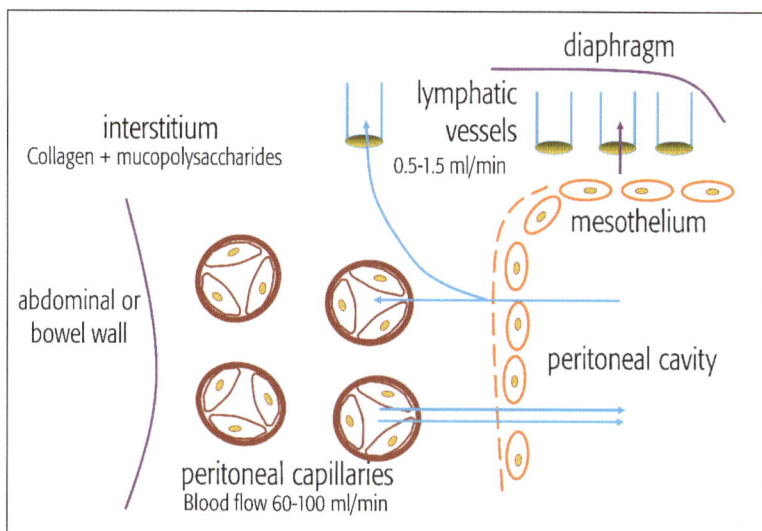

Figure 7.5. The Peritoneum as it Relates to Physiology of PD

PERITONEAL DIALYSIS ACCESS

A variety of silastic and polyurethane catheters are available for PD (reviewed in Chapter 5). The catheter can be placed laparoscopically or by open surgical technique. A double-cuff catheter with an arcuate subcutaneous tunnel and a caudad-oriented exit is recommended. It is best to wait 2 weeks before commencing PD to assure good healing and to prevent dialysate leaks (11,12).

PERITONEAL DIALYSIS FLUIDS

Conventional PD fluids consist of an aqueous solution of electrolytes similar to plasma, a bicarbonate precursor (usually lactate) and an osmotic agent, glucose for UF (13) (Table 7.1). Varied concentrations of dextrose (1.5%, 2.5%, 4.25%) are used to produce fluids of different osmolality. Glucose is widely accepted as an osmotic agent for PD because it is inexpensive and is considered relatively safe (at least until recently). One disadvantage is its small size. Consequently, it is rapidly absorbed into the blood with progressive loss of the osmotic gradient and long-term metabolic consequences, described below.

TABLE 7.1. Current PD Solutions (Baxter Corporation)

Solution Components	Solution PD1 Developed 1978	Solution PD2 Developed 1981	Solution PD4 Developed 1981
Dextrose (g/dl)	1.5, 2.5, 4.25	1.5, 2.5, 4.25	1.5, 2.5, 4.25
Sodium (mEq/L)	132.0	132.0	132.0
Chloride (mEq/L)	102.0	96.0	95.0
Calcium (mEq/L)	3.5	3.5	2.5
Magnesium (mEq/L)	1.5	0.5	0.5
Lactate (mEq/L)	35.0	40.0	40.0
Osmolality (mmol/L)	346–485	346–485	346–485
pH	5.2	5.2	5.2

PERITONEAL DIALYSIS SCHEDULES

Peritoneal dialysis can be done manually or with automated devices. It can be continuous (fluid in the abdominal cavity 24 hours a day) or intermittent (abdominal cavity dry for a part of the day). The latter being utilized in patients with considerable RRF. (Figure 7.6)

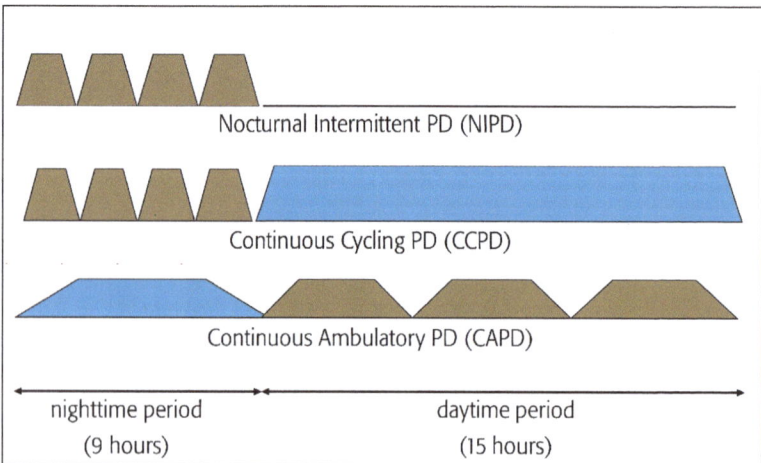

Figure 7.6. Peritoneal Dialysis Schedules

PHYSIOLOGY OF PERITONEAL DIALYSIS

In PD, the peritoneal membrane is utilized as an endogenous dialyzing membrane for removal of uremic toxins and excess fluid. Although various models of peritoneal membrane have been proposed, the three-pore model is most widely accepted to explain solute and water transport across the peritoneum (14–17). It assumes capillary endothelium to be the major barrier to solute and water transport, which ensues through a system of pores that can be classified into three broad categories, ultra small, small, and large pores (16–18). The abundant small pores (40–60 Å radii) are the tortuous intercellular clefts between the endothelial cells. The ultra-small pores (radius 3–5 Å), also present in a large number, are likely transendothelial aquaporin-1 (19–21). Additionally, a small number of large pores (200–300 Å radii) are present. Their nature remains unclear. (Figures 7.7 and 7.8)

Two major mechanisms, diffusion and convection (ultrafiltration), are involved in fluid and solute transport across the peritoneum (22).

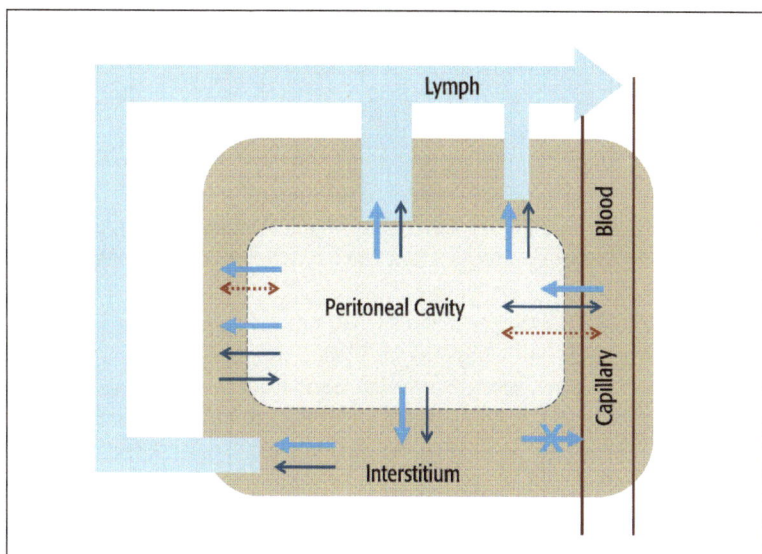

Figure 7.7. Water and Solute Transport across Peritoneal Membrane

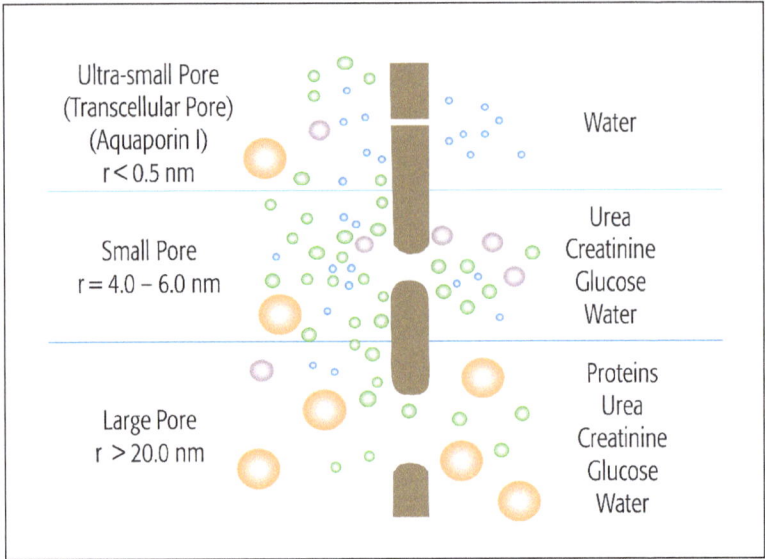

Figure 7.8. Three-pore Model of the Peritoneal Membrane

Diffusion, the most important transport mechanism for low molecular weight solutes, occurs through the small pore system (Figure 7.9). The permeability of the peritoneum to the transport of low molecular weight solutes is traditionally investigated by performing a standardized peritoneal equilibration test (PET), using a 4-hour exchange with 2.0 liters of 2.5% dextrose dialysate (23). The dialysate to plasma (D/P) ratio of creatinine at 4 hours is used to classify the peritoneum into 4 transport categories: Slow, Slow-average, Rapid-average, and Rapid (Table 7.2). Patients who exhibit rapid transport character will rapidly equilibrate creatinine and urea and achieve excellent small solute clearance. However, they will also rapidly absorb glucose from the peritoneal cavity and therefore swiftly lose osmotic gradient leading to poor UF. In contrast, patients who are slow transporters will have poor urea and creatinine clearance but excellent UF.

Ultrafiltration is achieved by using hypertonic glucose to create a crystalloid osmotic pressure gradient between the dialysate and the blood (24). The concentration of glucose is maximal at the beginning of dialysis but decreases during the dwell because of diffusion into blood across the small pores. Consequently, the UF rate is maximal at the start but decreases during the PD dwell. About 60% of the instilled glucose is absorbed during a 4-hour dwell. (Figures 7.10 and 7.11)

In addition to diffusion and convection, peritoneal fluid is being reabsorbed at a relatively constant rate of 1–1.5 ml/min, either directly into the sub-diaphragmatic lymphatics or into the interstitium and thereafter to lymphatics and post-capillary venules (24,25) (Figure 7.10).

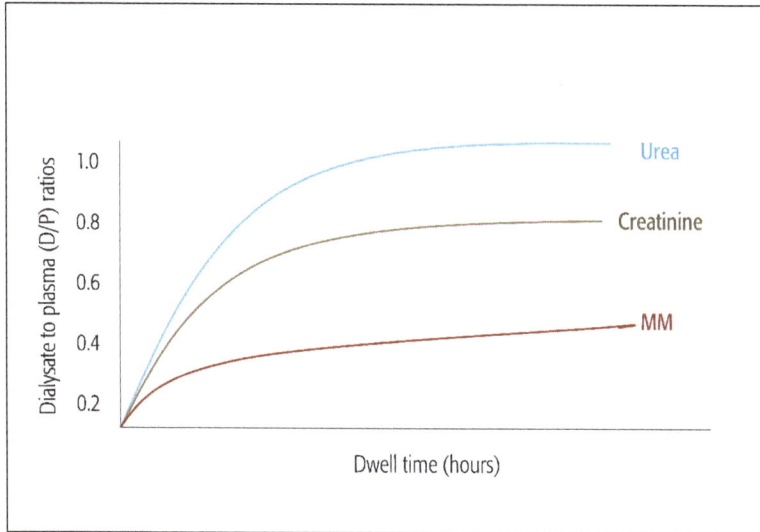

Figure 7.9. Theoretical Diffusion Curves for Various Solutes across the Peritoneal Membrane
(Daugirdas J, Blake P, Ing T, et al. *Handbook of Dialysis*, 3rd Ed. Philadelphia, PA, USA: Lippencott Williams & Wilkins; 2000; p 363)

TABLE 7.2. Membrane Classifications Using 2 L of 2.5% Dextrose at 4 Hours.

Membrane Classification	UF	D/P Creatinine
Rapid	(470) to 35	0.82–1.03
Rapid-Average	35 to 320	0.65–0.81
Slow-Average	320 to 600	0.5–0.64
Slow	600 to 1276	0.34–0.49

The number in parenthesis refers to negative UF. Abbreviation: UF, ultrafiltration; D/P, dialysate to plasma

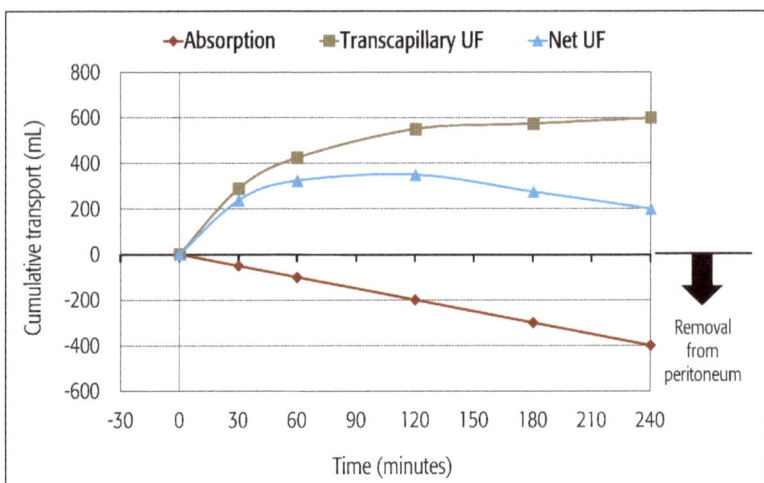

Figure 7.10. Net UF: Balance of Opposing Forces
(Mactier RA, Khanna R, Twardowski Z, et al. Contribution of lymphatic absorption to loss
of ultrafiltration and solute clearances in continuous ambulatory peritoneal dialysis. *J Clin
Invest* 1987; 80: 1311–1316.)

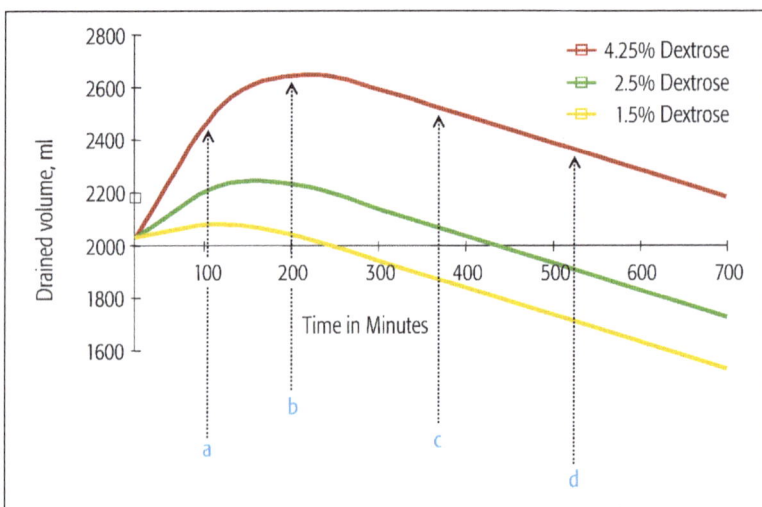

Figure 7.11. Determinants of UF Profile: Dextrose Strength, Duration, and Drain
Volume
(Rippe B, Stelin G, Haraldsson B. Computer simulations of peritoneal fluid transport in
CAPD. *Kidney Int* 1991; 40: 315-325.)

MARKERS OF PERITONEAL TRANSPORT

A number of substances present in the dialysis effluent are produced intrinsically by the peritoneal cells. Among these are various cytokines but also phospholipids, glycoproteins and glycosaminoglycans. The phospholipids in effluent largely consist of phosphatidylcholine (55–85%). They are mainly, but not exclusively, synthesized in mesothelial cells (26). Glycosaminoglycans, consisting of hyaluronans and proteoglycans, are also mainly, but not exclusively, synthesized in mesothelial cells (27,28). Cancer antigen 125(CA-125) is a 220 KD glycoprotein synthesized exclusively by mesothelial cells in the peritoneal tissue (29). The concentration of CA-125 in peritoneal effluent represents mesothelial cell mass in a stable PD patient (29–31). The following further supports this conclusion: 1. A positive relationship is present between the number of mesothelial cells and CA-125 level in the peritoneal effluent. 2. Cancer antigen 125 is not synthesized by other cells present in peritoneal tissue or by leukocytes (29–31).

During processing of procollagen I and III to collagen, procollagen I C terminal peptides (PICP) and procollagen III N terminal peptide (PIIINP) are split off. The dialysate concentration of PICP and PIIINP could be used as markers of collagen synthesis in the peritoneum (32).

PROS AND CONS OF PERITONEAL DIALYSIS

Peritoneal dialysis offers several advantages over HD. Unlike the interrupted, on-and-off treatment with HD, PD delivers a slow, steady treatment thereby avoiding wide fluctuations of plasma volume and solutes, and is generally better tolerated by patients with cardiovascular compromise. Additionally, PD provides a flexible schedule (unlike fixed HD shifts), thus bestowing patients opportunities to work, travel and participate in daytime activities. With PD being needleless, patients on PD do not have the anxiety experienced by patients on HD at the thought needle sticks. Avoiding needle sticks also helps to preserve arteriovenous access sites for future HD and minimize the risk of acquiring blood-borne infections like Hepatitis C. Additionally, PD facilitates preservation of RRF better than HD (33–39). Peritoneal dialysis may also be beneficial in patients waiting for kidney transplant. Recent data suggests that compared to HD, patients on PD have a significantly lower incidence of delayed graft function, a significantly lower requirement of dialysis in the post-transplant period, better long-term transplant outcomes, and better patient survival. Moreover, PD is less expensive per patient, per year than HD, with the difference estimated to be more than $20,000/patient/year, based on 2011 USRDS annual data report (1). (Table 1.3)

Notwithstanding the previously mentioned advantages, there are certain drawbacks of PD. Peritoneal dialysis is a continuous therapy with no "off" days and therefore may be inconvenient, leading to fatigue and burn-out of patients and families. Some patients may have concern with the body image resulting from the presence of a catheter and fluid in the abdomen. Moreover, there are minimal but finite risks of infections and mechanical complications like hernias, catheter leaks, and catheter malfunction.

RESIDUAL RENAL FUNCTION AND PERITONEAL DIALYSIS

The RRF progressively declines in virtually all patients, both before and after initiation of dialysis. There is ample clinical data to support that RRF declines more slowly in PD than in HD (33–35) (Figure 7.12). One possible explanation is that patients on PD have more hemodynamic stability with less abrupt volume and osmolar shifts. Furthermore, patients on PD are in a mild, constant volume expanded state with a relatively stable glomerular capillary pressure and minimal glomerular ischemia. Additionally, potential nephrotoxic inflammatory mediators generated by bioincompatible HD membranes are not observed in PD.

There is growing evidence that RRF is directly related to dialysis adequacy, conserved endocrine function, enhanced middle-molecule-clearance, better volume and blood-pressure control and superior survival outcomes (35,36,40,41) (Table 7.3).

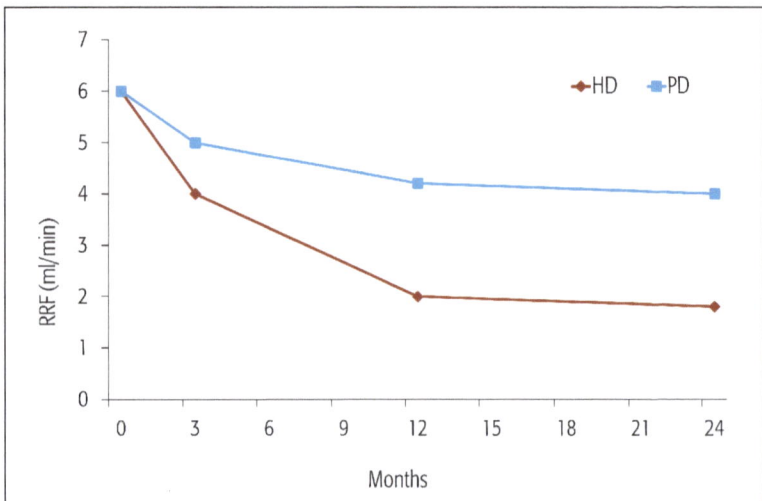

Figure 7.12. PD Preserves RRF Better than HD
(Lamiere N, Van Biesen W. *Perit Dial Int* 1997; 17 (suppl 2): 102-110)

Thus, preservation of RRF is an important goal in the management of patients on PD. Every effort should be made to avoid nephrotoxic drugs like aminoglycosides and non-steroidal anti-inflammatory drugs, and limit the use of radio-contrast agents (42,43). Use of angiotensin converting enzyme inhibitors (or angiotensin receptor blockers) may help to preserve RRF (44). Lastly, as PD preserves RRF better than HD, PD should be the modality of choice in patients with potentially reversible renal failure (45).

TABLE 7.3. Significance of RRF
Maintenance of endocrine functions
- EPO synthesis
- Activation of vitamin D
Elimination of b2 microglobulin/ middle molecules
- Lower risk of amyloidosis
Improved water and electrolyte balance
- Better BP control
- Decreased incidence of left ventricular hypertrophy
Improved survival
- Renal clearance more important than peritoneal clearance for survival

---

PERITONEAL DIALYSIS OUTCOME STUDIES

Earlier studies comparing the outcomes of the 2 modalities generally found similar mortality risks for patients on HD and PD (46–48). Thereafter a report based on the USRDS data of prevalent patients showed that patients on PD had a 19% higher mortality risk compared to patients on HD (49). This caused considerable concern in the USA. However, when a case-mix of USRDS incident and prevalent patients was subsequently analyzed, no difference in mortality between HD and PD was observed (50). Subsequent analysis of incident patients on dialysis from the Canadian, USA Medicare, and Danish registry data found a significantly lower relative risk of mortality in PD compared to HD in all groups of patients except elderly diabetic women (51–54). Interestingly, the lower mortality in PD was observed in the first 2 years of the treatment with no subsequent difference.

So far, studies comparing outcomes of PD with HD have been observational, based largely upon registry data. The mortality results from these studies should be viewed with caution since other unmeasured co-morbid factors and the severity of the reported co-morbidities may be unevenly distributed between the 2 groups and can lead to the difference observed in mortality risks between the 2 modalities. There is a great need for a randomized controlled trial, but the challenge to conduct one is underscored by the only

randomized controlled trial done hitherto (55). This multi-center Dutch trial
was discontinued prematurely because of poor enrollment. Notwithstanding
the small sample size, the study showed a significant survival benefit for PD
over HD in the first 4 years of the treatment.

Taken together, the results from the previously mentioned studies suggest that overall mortality is at least similar in HD and PD. Peritoneal dialysis
may offer survival benefit in the first 2 years of the treatment. There may be a
higher risk of mortality among elderly diabetic female patients on PD, which
may, in turn, be related to higher prevalence of coronary artery disease and
congestive heart failure in such a population (56,57). (Figures 7.13–7.17)

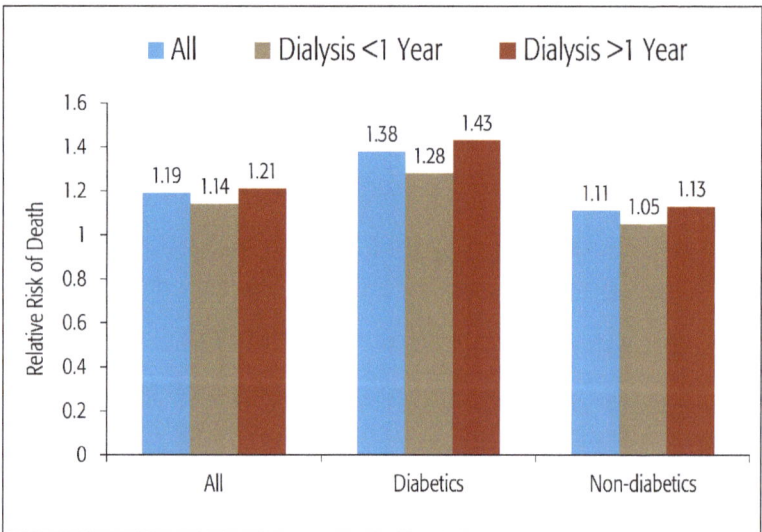

Figure 7.13. Relative Risk of Death in Dialysis Patients
The relative risk of death is higher in prevalent PD patients. (Bloembergen WE, Port FK,
Mauger EA, et al. A comparison of mortality between patients treated with hemodialysis
and peritoneal dialysis. *J Am Soc Nephrol* 1995; 6: 177-83.)

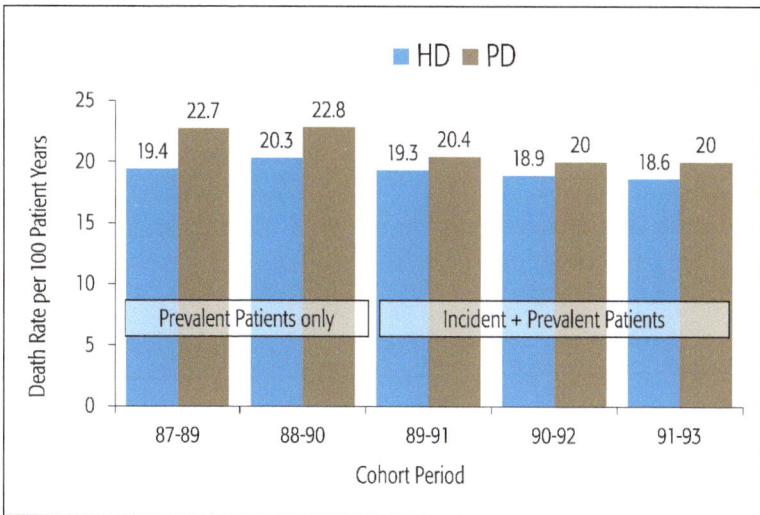

Figure 7.14. Trends in Adjusted All-cause Death Rates for HD and PD Patients USRDS cohorts from the 1990 decade. (Vonesh EF, Moran J. Mortality in end-stage renal disease: A reassessment of differences between patients treated with hemodialysis and peritoneal dialysis. *J Am Soc Nephrol* 1999; 10: 354-65.)

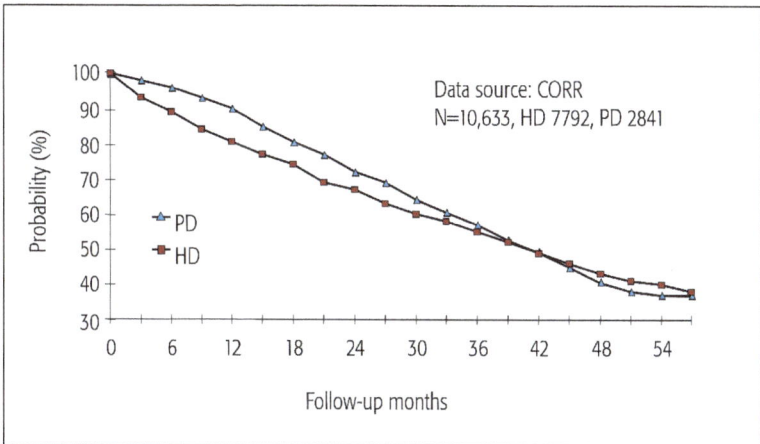

Figure 7.15. Survival Probability for Patients Initiating Dialysis with PD Compared to HD (1990–94)
(Fenton SSA, Schaubel DE, Desmeules M, et al. Hemodialysis versus peritoneal dialysis: A comparison of adjusted mortality rates. *Am J Kid Dis* 1997; 30: 334-42.)

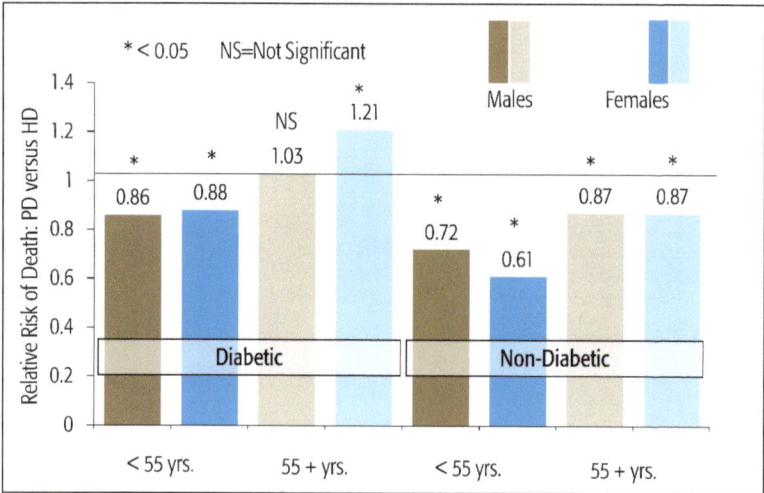

Figure 7.16. Relative Risk of Death in PD versus HD Patients
All incident Medicare patients 1994–96; follow-up through 1997; adjusted for age, gender, race, cause of ESRD. (Collins AJ, Hao W, Xia H, et al. Mortality risks of peritoneal dialysis and hemodialysis. *Am J Kid Dis* 1999; 34: 1065-74.9)

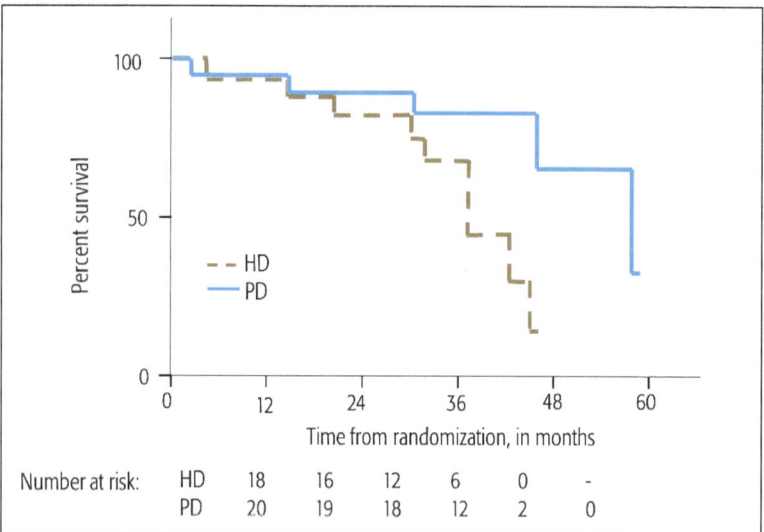

Figure 7.17. Randomized Controlled Study Comparing Survival in HD versus PD
(Korevaar JC, Feith GW, Dekker FW, et al. Effect of starting with hemodialysis compared with peritoneal dialysis in patients new on dialysis treatment: A randomized controlled trial. *Kidney Int* 2003; 64: 2222-28.)

CURRENT PROBLEMS WITH PERITONEAL DIALYSIS

Although PD may provide a superior mode of dialysis to HD, the benefits of PD are limited to the first 2–4 years with the majority of patients shifting to HD because of technique failure. The PD technique survival is 30–50% at 5 years and is less than 20% at 10 years (58,59). Causes of treatment failure include recurrent episodes of peritonitis, loss of RRF (Figure 7.18), inadequate solute clearance, and loss of peritoneal membrane function (58–60). With innovation in PD techniques, there have been significant improvements in peritonitis rate and solute clearance. However, 1 major cause of long-term PD nonachievement that remains unaddressed is related to the ongoing peritoneal structural and functional changes leading to membrane failure.

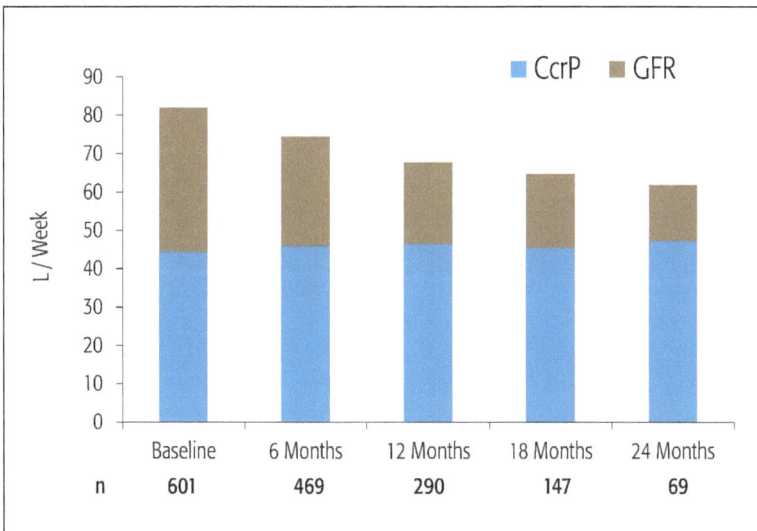

Figure 7.18. Residual Renal Function and Peritoneal Creatinine Clearance over Time Abbreviations: CcrP, clearance of creatinine from plasma; GFR, glomerular filtration rate; L, liters; n, number of subjects at each timeline. (Bargman JM, Thorpe KE, Churchill DN. Relative contribution of RRF and peritoneal clearance of adequacy of dialysis: A reanalysis of CANUSA study. *J Am Soc Nephrol* 2001; 12: 2158-62.)

STRUCTURAL CHANGES IN THE PERITONEAL MEMBRANE DURING PERITONEAL DIALYSIS

Compilation of data from peritoneal biopsy series suggests that long-term PD is associated with progressive morphologic changes in the various components of the peritoneal membrane (61). Alteration of mesothelial pheno-type with gradual loss of microvilli, separation of intercellular junction and eventual loss of mesothelial cells is seen as early as 3 months on PD (62). Concurrently, there is a gradual increase in the thickness of sub-mesothelial interstitium due to edema and increased collagen deposition (61). In addition, there is an increase in the number of interstitial cells, which may represent mesenchymal cells entrapped in the interstitial stroma or alternatively, transdifferentiated mesothelial cells and are likely involved in the peritoneal fibrosis (62,63).

Changes in peritoneal vasculature parallel mesothelial and interstitial alteration and include reduplication of the capillary basement lamina and later fusion of these layers to give the appearance of a thickened membrane. The thickness of the capillary membrane increases as dialysis goes on, until the capillary is completely occluded (61,62). Moreover, the number of blood vessels per unit length of the peritoneal surface also increases with the duration of PD (62).

FUNCTIONAL CHANGES IN THE PERITONEAL MEMBRANE WITH LONG-TERM PERITONEAL DIALYSIS

There is mounting evidence that with time, UF capacity of peritoneal membrane is progressively lost with concomitant increase in the peritoneal small solute transport rate (58,64,65) (Figure 7.19). The upsurge in small solute transport reflects an increase in effective peritoneal surface area due to proliferation of capillaries (neoangiogenesis).

Altered peritoneal membrane functions have a significant impact on both technique and patient survival (58,61–65) (Figure 7.20). As prevalence of UF failure increases, it becomes the predominant reason for drop out among patients on PD for a long period of time (59). Reduced UF capacity leads to a chronic volume overload state with resultant congestive heart failure and cardiovascular mortality (66–68). Poor UF can also lead to low drain volumes and consequently to poor solute clearance and thus lower dialysis adequacy. In addition, patients with UF failure experience rapid absorption of glucose from the dialysate (with inhibition of appetite) and a greater loss of proteins in the dialysate leading to poor nutritional status and adverse outcomes (66–68).

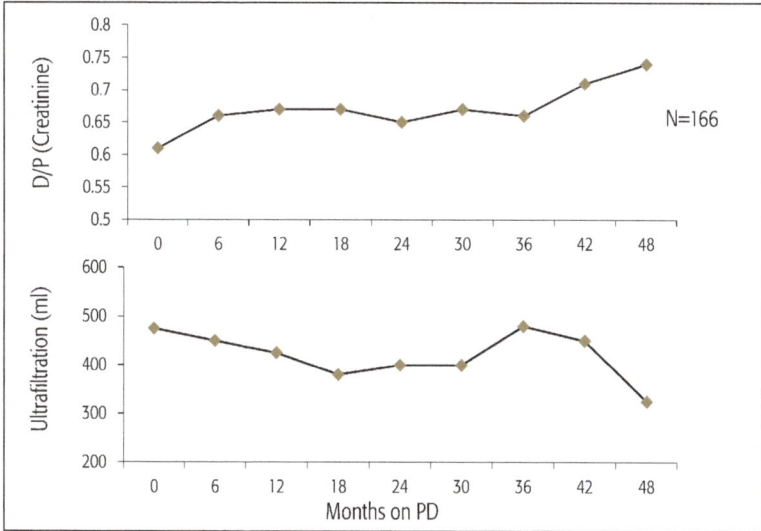

Figure 7.19. Longitudinal Changes in Peritoneal Permeability and UF
Abbreviation: D/P, dialysate to plasma ratio. (Davies S, Bryan J, Phillips L, et al. Longitudinal changes in peritoneal kinetics: The effect of peritoneal dialysis and peritonitis. *Nephrol Dial Transplant* 1996; 11: 498-506.)

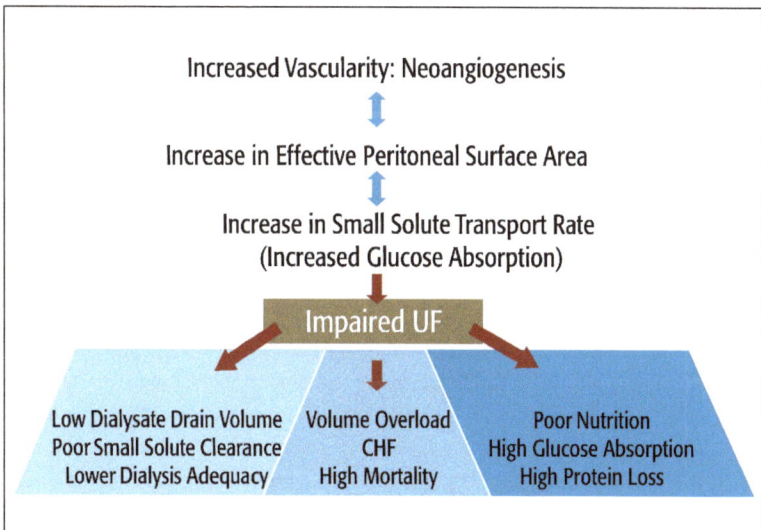

Figure 7.20. Consequences of Structural/Functional Changes in the Peritoneal Membrane with Long-term PD

Potential Causative Factors for Peritoneal Membrane Changes in Long-term Peritoneal Dialysis

During PD, the peritoneum is continuously exposed to non-physiologic dialysis solutions, which are hyperosmolar, acidic, and have high glucose and lactate content. Additionally, during heat sterilization and storage of the dialysate, glucose is degraded to reactive substances called glucose degradation products (GDPs). Any of the previously mentioned elements can be potentially toxic to the peritoneal membrane.

Low pH

Conventional PD solutions have a pH of 5.2 and a lactate concentration of 40 mmol/L. Infusion pain is the most direct and immediate clinical consequence of low pH (69, 70). Furthermore, in vitro studies have demonstrated the toxic effects of low pH and lactate on mesothelial cells and peritoneal host defense (71). Raising the pH of dialysate to 6.5 or higher prevents impairment of various cell functions and diminution of infusion pain (69,70,72,73).

Glucose

To be effective as an osmotic agent, the glucose concentrations must typically be 15–40 times physiological levels (1370–3860 mg/dL). Consequently, glucose is absorbed into blood and may be associated with metabolic problems such as hyperglycemia, hyperinsulinemia, hyperlipidemia and obesity (74,75). Furthermore, glucose may also influence cell functions through hyperosmolarity, GDPs, and reactions mediated by advanced glycation end-products (AGEs). Experimental evidence suggests that glucose may be toxic to the peritoneal mesothelial cells and leukocytes (76,77). Moreover, increase in the rate of fibroblast proliferation and collagen synthesis and up regulation of vascular endothelial growth factor synthesis by glucose suggests that it may play a direct role in peritoneal fibrosis and neoangiogenesis (76–79).

Glucose Degradation Products

During heat sterilization and storage, some glucose in the PD fluid is degraded to highly reactive substances referred to as GDPs (80). The presence and toxicity of GDPs in PD fluids has been well demonstrated in experimental studies (81,82). Although all GDPs are highly reactive carbonyl compounds of small molecular weight, known to be extremely toxic (Table 7.4), the recently identified 3, 4-DGE, is reported to be the most biologically active of all GDPs identified so far (83,84). The presence of GDPs in PD fluid seems to be a major factor responsible for mesothelial cell loss observed during the course of PD (85–87). Apart from their inherent toxic effects, it is now recognized that GDPs are much stronger promoters of AGEs than glucose per se. AGEs are known to accumulate over time and are considered to participate in remodeling and fibrosis of the peritoneal membrane (88). (Table 7.4)

TABLE 7.4. GDPs and their Concentrations in Glucose and Icodextrin-based PD Solutions

Compound	Formula	Concentration Glucose-based Solutions	mmol/L Icodextrin
Acetaldehyde	C2H4O	120–420	35
3-DG	C6H10O5	47–118	4
Formaldehyde	CH2O	4.6–15	ND
2-Furaldehyde	C5H4O2	0.05–2	ND
Glyoxal	C2H2O2	3.0–14	2.6
5-HMF	C6H6O3	2.2–30	ND
Methylglyoxal	C3H4O3	2.0–22.7	1.9

Abbreviation: ND, Not Determined. (Cooker LA, Holmes CJ, Hoff CM. Biocompatibility of icodextrin. Kidney Int 2002; 62 (suppl 81): S34-45.)

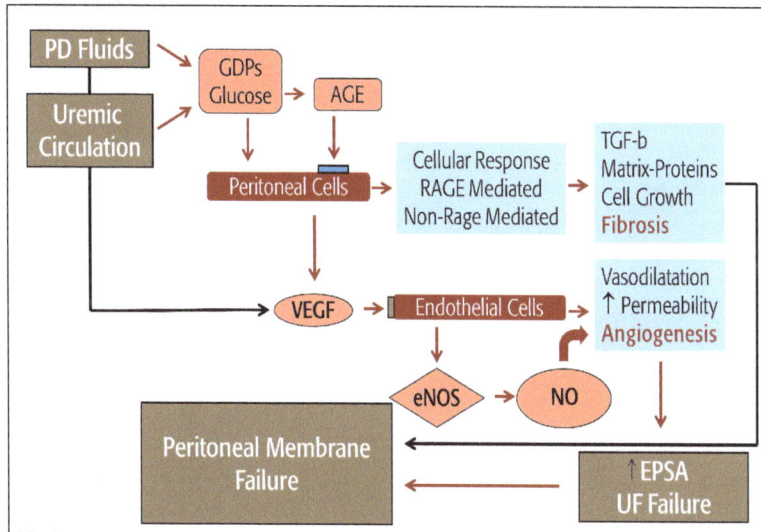

Figure 7.21. Theory of Peritoneal Membrane Dysfunction in Long-term PD
Abbreviations: AGE, advanced glycation end-products; eNos, endothelial nitric oxide synthase; EPSA, effective peritoneal surface area; GPD, glucose degradation products; NO, nitric oxide; RAGE, receptor for AGE; TGF-b, transforming growth factor-beta; VEGF, vascular endothelial growth factor.

Advanced Glycation End-Products

Glucose can also contribute indirectly to peritoneal membrane alterations through formation of AGEs (89,90). Advanced glycation end-products have been implicated in various activities that can adversely affect the peritoneal membrane, including protein cross-linking, inflammation, angiogenesis, vascular smooth muscle proliferation, and increased nitric oxide production (91–93). A recent histochemical analysis of peritoneal membrane biopsy demonstrated co-localization of AGEs with TGF-β, VEGF, and M-CSF, suggesting that AGE-receptor binding activates signaling pathways leading to development of peritoneal fibrosis and neovascularization (94). Furthermore, AGEs have been shown to reduce the mesothelial cell viability and increase VCAM-1 and plasminogen activator inhibitor-1 (PAI-1) expression in mesothelial cells (95,96). Thus, AGEs play a significant role in peritoneal membrane alteration in long-term PD. (Figure 7.21)

How Can Glucose Degradation Products Be Avoided?

It is well known that pH, glucose concentration, and presence of catalyzing substances affect degradation. For a standard PD solution, hydrochloric acid is added to reach pH 5.0-5.5, and although GDPs are still formed, the compromise has for many years been considered satisfactory. Further lowering of pH has not been possible because of poor tolerance due to infusion pain and compromise of host defense. Recently, multi-compartment bags have been developed in which 1 compartment contains a very high concentration of glucose (50%) with very low pH (3.2) while the other compartment contains the buffer and other electrolytes (97). When the PD fluid is heat sterilized in compartmentalized bags, few GDPs are generated. Mixing the fluids of the compartments just prior to infusion results in a final solution with a pH close to the physiologic value (7.4) and a minimal GDP concentration.

Another approach to avoid GDPs is to sterilize the solution without heat, using stepwise ultrafilters, to remove bacteria and pyrogens. Some GDPs are still generated. This method is not yet in commercial use (98).

Finally, an obvious approach would be to avoid using glucose and to select alternative osmotic agents. Among alternative agents available today or in clinical trials, no candidate has appeared to replace glucose completely. Amino acids and icodextrins are indicated in certain cases but usually for only 1 dwell per day (99). In addition, icodextrin, being a glucose polymer, also contains some GDPs after heat sterilization.

NEW SOLUTIONS FOR PERITONEAL DIALYSIS

Three new PD solutions have been recently introduced for clinical use in Europe. They offer significant advancement in the acute and chronic effects of bioincompatible PD solutions such as infusion pain, loss of UF, impaired host defense, malnutrition and technique failure.

Icodextrin-Based Solution

Icodextrin is a large polymer of glucose (16KD) produced by the hydrolysis of cornstarch, and consists of glucose units linked predominantly by α 1–4 glucosidic bonds (100). Icodextrin 7.5% PD solution is iso-osmolar to plasma (284 mOsm/kg), and employs colloidal, rather than crystalloid, osmotic pressure to yield a sustained UF profile that is equivalent to, or better than that of 4.25% dextrose solution. Long-term clinical experience with icodextrin now extends over many years in Europe, and icodextrin has been demonstrated to extend PD technique survival in patients with UF failure (101). It is more biocompatible to the peritoneum than glucose because it is iso-osmolar, has low GDPs concentration, and demonstrates a significant reduction in cell cytotoxicity and AGE formation (102). Icodextrin usage is accompanied by a sustained, reversible rise in plasma oligosaccharides, particularly maltose, though no clinical adverse effects have been reported even after several years of continuous use. A decline in serum amylase level due to interference by icodextrin metabolites on amylase assay has been observed and it is therefore recommended not to rely on serum amylase alone in diagnosing pancreatitis in patients on icodextrin. Some adverse effects, especially reversible skin reactions (2.5%), have been reported (101). Icodextrin was recently approved by the FDA for use in long dwells for patients with rapid and rapid-average transport characteristics. (Figures 7.22 and 7.23; Table 7.5)

Peritoneal dialysis solutions are packaged in bags with color-coded connection devices, designed for convenience and safety, indicating the various concentrations of dextrose (Figure 7.24).

TABLE 7.5. An Iso-osmolar Formulation: Icodextrin versus Conventional PD Solution

Solution Components	ICODEXTRIN	CONVENTIONAL
Dextrose (g/dL)	—	1.5, 2.5, 4.25
Icodextrin (g/dL)	7.5	—
Sodium (mEq/L)	132	132
Chloride (mEq/L)	96	96
Calcium (mEq/L)	1.75	1.75
Magnesium (mEq/L)	0.5	0.5
Lactate (mEq/L)	40	40
Osmolality (mOsm/kg)	282–286	346–485
pH	5.2	5.2

Solutions Containing Amino Acids

Peritoneal dialysis is associated with a daily peritoneal effluent loss of 6–9 g of protein and 1–2 g of amino acids (103). Various solutions containing amino acids have been proposed as alternative osmotic agents to glucose to potentially improve nitrogen balance and concurrently reduce the glucose load. Peritoneal dialysis solutions containing amino acids are not available in the USA, but a solution with 1.1% amino acids is now commercially available in Europe. One exchange with a 1.1% solution results in the absorption of about 13–20 g of amino acids (104). Solutions containing amino acids also improve biocompatibility as they lack glucose and GDPs and have more physiologic pH (7.2). However, the use of solutions containing amino acids can result in azotemia and metabolic acidosis. Therefore, only 1 or a maximum of 2 daily exchanges of solution containing 1.1% amino acids are recommended (104).

Bicarbonate-Buffered Solutions

Recently, multi-compartment bags (Figure 7.25) have been developed to minimize GDP formation and have bicarbonate buffer with physiologic pH. One chamber contains glucose at a very high concentration (50% dextrose), calcium chloride and magnesium chloride at a pH of 3.5, while the other chamber contains sodium chloride and sodium bicarbonate with or without lactate. Mixing of the 2 fluids just prior to infusion results in a final solution with a pH close to the physiologic value (7.4) and a minimal GDP concentration (97,105,106). Clinical and experimental studies indicate that the control of acidosis is at least as good as that with conventional PD solutions and that the new solutions may have a favorable impact on peritoneal membrane integrity (97,105–107). Multi-chambered solutions are not available in the USA but have recently been introduced in Europe (Table 7.6 and Figure 7.26)

TABLE 7.6. Dialysate Composition

Component	HD	Conventional	Dual-chambered
Sodium (mM)	135–155	132	132
Potassium (mM)	0–4.0	0	0
Calcium (mM)	0–2.0	1.25–1.75	1.25–1.75
Magnesium (mM)	0–0.75	0.25–0.75	0.25
Chloride (mM)	87–120	95–96	95–96
Dextrose (g/dl)	0–0.20	1.5–4.25	1.5–4.25
Bicarbonate (mM)	25–40	–	25
Lactate (mM)	–	35–40	15

(Pastan S, Bailey J. *N Engl J Med* 1998; 338:1428–1437)

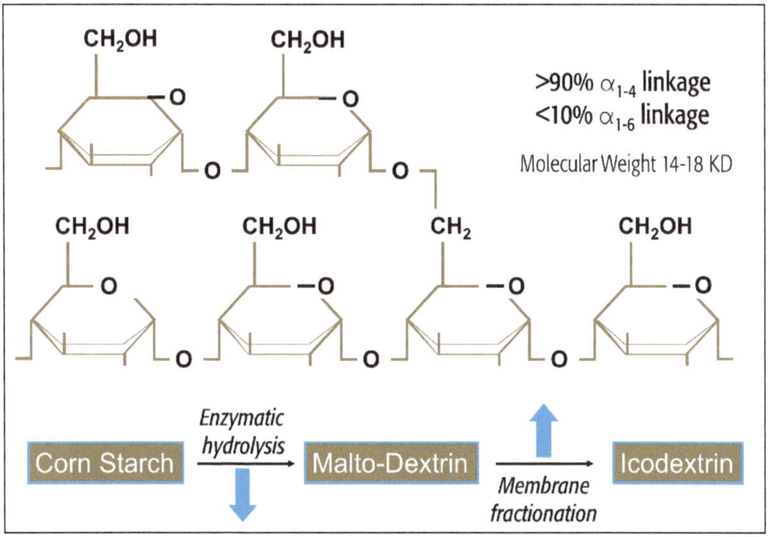

Figure 7.22. Icodextrin: A High Molecular Weight Glucose Polymer

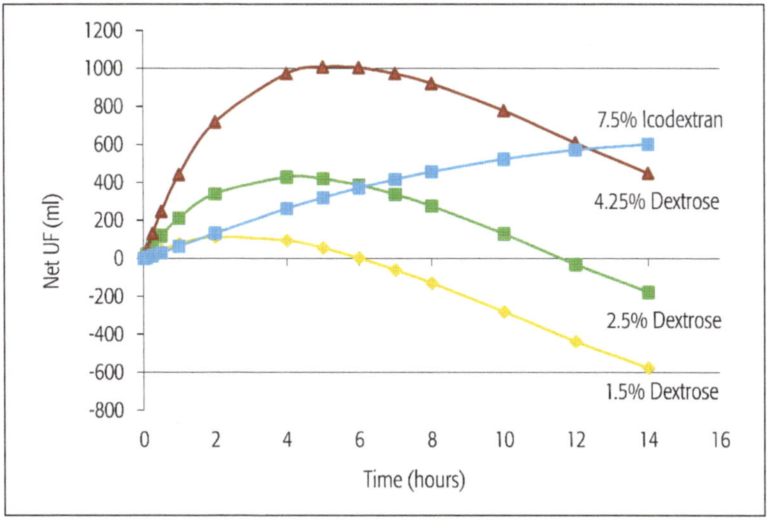

Figure 7.23. Dextrose versus Icodextrin net UF
(Ho-dac-Pannekeet MM, Schouten N, Langendijk MJ, et al. Peritoneal transport characteristics with glucose polymer based dialysate. *Kid Int* 1996; 50;979-86. Douma C, Hiralall J, de Waart D, Struijk DG, Krediet R. Icodextrin with notroprusside increases ultrafiltration and peritoneal transport during long CAPD dwells. *Kid Int* 1998; 53:1014–1021.)

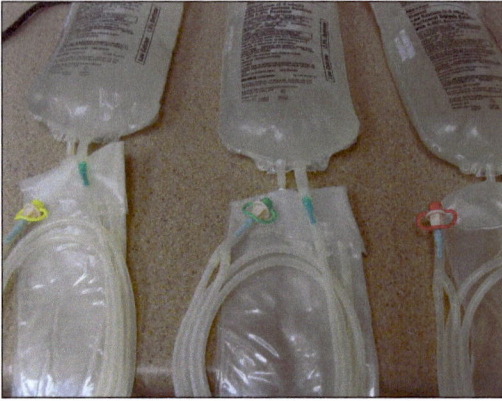

Figure 7.24. Dialysis Solution Bags
The color-coded connection devices indicate the
concentration of dextrose: yellow = 1.5%, green = 2.5%,
and red = 4.5%. These color codes are also used to
illustrate the dextrose concentrations in Figures 7.11 and
7.23.

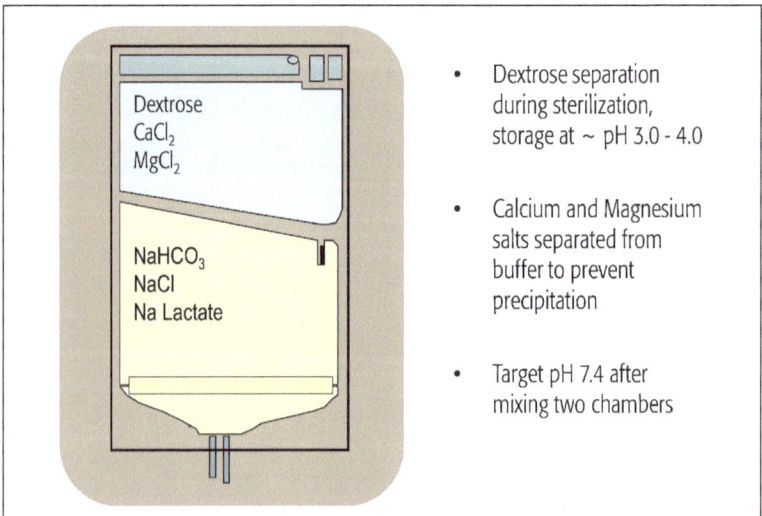

- Dextrose separation
  during sterilization,
  storage at ~ pH 3.0 - 4.0

- Calcium and Magnesium
  salts separated from
  buffer to prevent
  precipitation

- Target pH 7.4 after
  mixing two chambers

Dextrose
$CaCl_2$
$MgCl_2$

$NaHCO_3$
NaCl
Na Lactate

Figure 7.25. Dual-chambered Bicarbonate Dialysate

FUTURE STRATEGY FOR USE OF PERITONEAL DIALYSIS SOLUTIONS

No currently available PD solution meets all requirements of an ideal solution: effective UF, long-term preservation of peritoneal membrane, and correction of nutritional and metabolic abnormalities. However, using the new PD solutions in combination may help to achieve these goals. Preliminary evidence suggests that a combination of 2 or all of the 3 new solutions provides equal or superior efficacy to standard glucose regimens and may protect the peritoneal membrane from the toxic effects of glucose and GDPs (108–111). Long-term prospective studies are needed to compare the efficacy of a combination of new PD solutions (Icodextrin for the long dwell, 1 dwell of amino acid solution and remaining dwells with bicarbonate/lactate solution) with a conventional glucose/lactate based solution. (Figure 7.26)

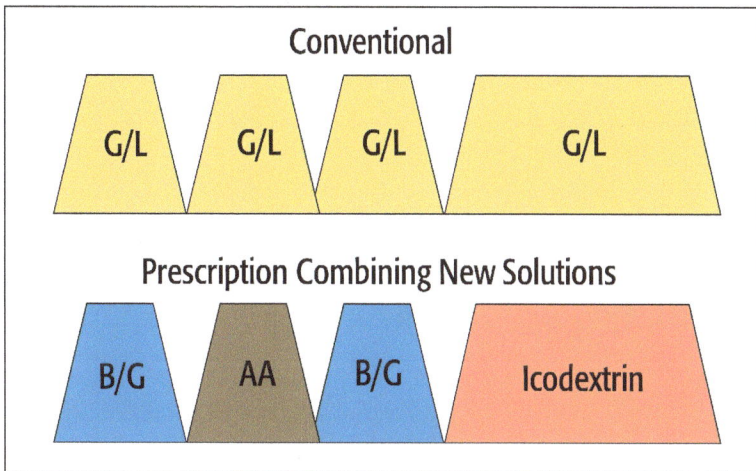

Figure 7.26. Conventional and Alternative Prescription Treatments
Abbreviations: AA, amino acid; B, bicarbonate; G, glucose; L, lactate.

LONG-TERM PROSPECTS

While the novel PD solutions offer an improvement in the biocompatibility, they do not completely abolish the formation of GDPs and their long-term effect on the peritoneum is not yet known. Identification of putative molecular mechanisms by which GDPs and AGEs initiate a number of cellular responses including increased expression of VEGF and TGF-β and interaction of VEGF with eNOS and NO to stimulate angiogenesis, evoke new therapeutic strategies that might protect the peritoneal membrane against the consequences of long-term PD. Modulating angiogenesis, inhibiting AGE formation, inhibiting L-arginine-NO pathway and finally gene therapy to reduce the levels of GDPs offer exciting new approaches to preserve the peritoneal membrane (112–114). It remains to be seen if these maneuvers will prove clinically beneficial. (Table 7.7)

TABLE 7.7. Potential Therapeutic Strategies to Protect the Peritoneal Membrane against Consequences of Long-Term PD
Reduction of Reactive Carbonyl Compounds
- Icodextrin
- Amino acid PD fluids
- Dual chambered / low GDP solutions

Inhibitors of AGE
- Aminoguanidine. Risk of neurotoxicity

Inhibition of L-arginine-NO pathway
- Compete binding of L-arginine to NOS: L-NAME

Modulate Angiogenesis
- Interference with VGEF
- Interference with receptor binding
- Interfere with endothelial cell adhesion and migration

REFERENCES

1.   United States Renal Data System, *Annual Data Report 2011*, Bethesda. MD

2.   Stack AG. Determinants of modality selection among incident dialysis patients: Results from a national study. *J Am Soc Nephrol* 2002; 13: 1279–1287.

3.   Mehrotra R, Blake P, Berman N, Nolph KD. An analysis of dialysis training in the United States and Canada. *Am J Kidney Dis* 2002; 40: 152–160.

4.   Kutner NG, Zhang R, Huang Y, Wasse H. Patient awareness and initiation of peritoneal dialysis [published online September 27, 2010]. *Arch Intern Med* doi: 10.1001/archinternmed.2010.361.

5.   Golper T. Patient education: can it maximize the success of therapy? *Nephrol Dial Transplant* 2001; 16 (Suppl 7) 20–4.

6.   Lo WK, Li FK, Choy CB, et al. A retrospective survey of attitudes towards acceptance of peritoneal dialysis in Chinese end stage renal failure patients in Hong Kong—From a cultural point of view. *Perit Dial Int* 2001; 21: S318–S321.

7.   Little J, Irwin A, Marshall T, Rayner H, Smith S. Predicting a patient's choice of dialysis modality: Experience in a United Kingdom renal department. *Am J Kidney Dis* 2001; 37: 981–986.

8. Dobbie JW. From philosopher to fish: Comparitive anatomy of the peritoneal cavity as an excretory organ and its significance for peritoneal dialysis in man. *Perit Dial Int* 1988; 8: 4–8.

9. Dobbie JW, Lloyd JK, Gall CA. Categorization of ultrastructural changes in peritoneal mesothelium, stroma and blood vessels in uremia and CAPD patients. *Adv Perit Dial* 1990; 6: 3–12.

10. Nagy JA. Peritoneal morphology and function. *Kidney Int* 1996; 50 (suppl 56): S2–11.

11. Gokal R, Alexander S, Ash S, et al. Peritoneal catheters and exit site practices toward optimum peritoneal access. 1998 update. *Perit Dial Int* 18: 11–33.

12. Figueiredo A, Goh BK, Jenkins S, et al. Clinical practice guidelines for peritoneal access. *Perit Dial Int* 2010; 30: 424–429.

13. Feriani M. Use of different buffers in peritoneal dialysis. *Semin Dialysis* 2000; 13: 256–60.

14. Dedrick RL, Flessner MF, Schultz JS. Is peritoneum a membrane? *Am Soc Artif Intern Organs trans* 1982; 5, 1–6.

15. Flessner MF, Dedrick RL, Schultz JS. A distributed model of peritoneal-plasma transport: theoretical considerations. *Am J Physiol* 1984; 246 R597–607.

16. Rippe B, Stelin G. Simulations of peritoneal solute transport during continuous ambulatory peritoneal dialysis (CAPD). Application of two-pore formulation. *Kidney Int* 1989; 35: 1234–1244.

17. Rippe B, Stelin G, Haraldsson B. Computer simulations of peritoneal fluid transport in CAPD. *Kidney Int* 1991; 40: 315–325.

18. Flessner MF. Osmotic barrier of the parietal peritoneum. Am J Physiol 1994; 267: F861–70.

19. Agre P, Preston BM, Smith BL, et al. Aquaporin CHIP: the archetypal molecular water channel. *Am J Physiol* 1993; 34: F463–476.

20. Pannekeet MM, Mulder JB, Weening JJ, et al. Demonstration of aquaporin-CHIP in peritoneal tissue of uremic and CAPD patients. *Perit Dial Int* 1996; 16 (suppl 1): S54–57.

21. Lai KN, Lam MF, Leung JC. Peritoneal function: The role of aquaporins. *Perit Dial Int* 2003; 23 (suppl 2): S20–25.

22. Leypoldt JK. Solute transport across the peritoneal membrane. *J Am Soc Nephrol* 2002; 13: S84–91.

23. Twardowski ZJ, Nolph KD, Khanna R, et al. Peritoneal equilibration test. *Perit Dial Bull* 1987; 7: 138–147.

24. Kreidet RT, Lindholm B, Rippe B. Pathophysiology of peritoneal membrane failure. *Perit Dial Int* 2000; 20 (suppl 4) S22–42.

25. Mactier RA, Khanna R, Twardowski Z, Moore H, Nolph KD. Contribution of lymphatic absorption to loss of ultrafiltration and solute clearances in continuous ambulatory peritoneal dialysis. *J Clin Invest* 1987; 80: 1311–1316.

26. Beavis J, Harwood JL, Coles GA, Williams JD. Synthesis of phospholipids by human peritoneal mesothelial cells. *Perit Dial Int* 1994; 14: 348–355.

27. Yung S, Thomas GJ, Stylianou E, et al. Source of peritoneal proteoglycans: Human peritoneal mesothelial cells synthesize and secrete mainly small dermatan sulfate proteoglycans. *Am J Pathol* 1995; 146: 520–529.

28. Yung S, Coles GA, Williams JD, Davies M. The source and possible significance of hyaluronans in peritoneal cavity. *Kidney Int* 1994; 46: 527–533.

29. Koomen GCM, Betjes MGH, Zemel D, Kreidet RT, Hoek FJ. Cancer antigen 125 is locally produced in the peritoneal cavity during continuous ambulatory peritoneal dialysis. *Perit Dial Int* 1994; 14: 132–136.

30. Visser CE, Brouwer SJJE, Betjes MGH, et al. Cancer antigen 125: A bulk marker for the mesothelial mass in stable peritoneal dialysis patients. *Nephrol Dial Transplant* 1995; 10: 64–69.

31. Pannekeet MM, Koomen GCM, Struijk, et al. Longitudinal follow-up of CA 125 in peritoneal effluent. *Kidney Int* 1997; 51: 888–893.

32. Joffe P, Jensen LT. Type I and III procollagens in CAPD: Markers of peritoneal fibrosis. *Adv Perit Dial* 1991; 7: 158–160.

33. Lameire N, Van Biesen W. The impact of residual renal function on the adequacy of peritoneal dialysis. *Perit Dial Int* 1997; 17 (suppl 2): S102–S110.

34. Jansen MA, Hart AA, Korevaar, JC, et al. Pedictor of rate of decline of residual renal function in incident dialysis patients. *Kidney Int* 2002; 62: 1046–53.

35. Bargman JM, Thorpe KE, Churchill DN. Relative contribution of residual renal function and peritoneal clearance of adequacy of dialysis: A reanalysis of the CANUSA study. *J Am Soc Nephrol* 2001; 12: 2158–62.

36. Paniagua R, Amato D, Vonesh E, et al. Effects of increased peritoneal clearances on mortality rates in peritoneal dialysis: ADEMEX, a prospective randomized controlled trial. *J Am Soc Nephrol* 2002; 13: 1307–20.

37. Bleyer AJ, Burkart JM, Russell GB, Adams PL. Dialysis modality and delayed graft function after cadaveric renal transplantation. *J Am Soc Nephrol* 1999; 10: 154–159.

38. Perez-Fontan M, Rodriguez CA, Garcia FT, et al. Delayed graft function after renal transplantation in patients undergoing peritoneal dialysis and hemodialysis. *Adv Perit Dial* 1996; 12: 101–104.

39. Miklos Z, Molnar MZ, Mehrotra R, et al. Dialysis Modality and Outcomes in Kidney Transplant Recipients Clin *J Am Soc Nephrol* 2012; 7: 332–341.

40. Churchill DN, Taylor DW, Keshaviah PR, et al. Adequacy of dialysis and nutrition in continuous peritoneal dialysis: Association with clinical outcomes. *J Am Soc Nephrol* 1996; 7: 198–207.

41. McCusker FX, Teehan BP, Thorpe KE, et al. How much peritoneal dialysis is required for the maintenance of a good nutritional state? *Kidney Int* 1996; 50 (supp 56): S56–61.

42. Singhal MK, Bhaskaran S, Vidgne E, et al. Rate of decline of residual renal function in patients on continuous peritoneal dialysis and factors affecting it. *Perit Dial Int* 2000; 20: 429–38.

43. Kim DJ, Park JA, Huh W, et al. The effect of hemodialysis during break-in period on residual renal function in CAPD patients. *Perit Dial Int* 2000; 20: 784–801.

44. Li PK-T, Chow K-M, Wong TY-H, et al. Effects of an angiotensin-converting enzyme inhibitor on residual renal function in patients receiving peritoneal dialysis. A randomized controlled study. *Ann Int Med* 2003; 139: 105–12.

45. Goldstein A, Kliger AS, Finkelstein FO. Recovery of renal function and the discontinuation of dialysis in patients treated with continuous peritoneal dialysis. *Perit Dial Int* 2003; 23: 151–6.

46. Maiorca R, Vonesh E, Cancarini, et al. A six year comparison of patient and technique survivals in CAPD and HD. *Kidney Int* 1988; 34: 518–24.

47. Burton PR, Walls JA. A selection adjusted comparison of hospitalization on continuous ambulatory peritoneal dialysis and hemodialysis: 4-year analysis of a prospective multicenter study. *Lancet* 1987; ii: 1105–9.

48. Wolfe RA, Port FK, Hawthorne VM, Guire KE. A comparison of survival among dialytic therapies of choice: in-center hemodialysis versus continuous ambulatory peritoneal dialysis at home. *Am J Kid Dis* 1990; 15: 433–40.

49. Bloembergen WE, Port FK, Mauger EA, Wolfe RA. A comparison of mortality between patients treated with hemodialysis and peritoneal dialysis. *J Am Soc Nephrol* 1995; 6: 177–83.

50. Vonesh EF, Moran J. Mortality in end-stage renal disease: A reassessment of differences between patients treated with hemodialysis and peritoneal dialysis. *J Am Soc Nephrol* 1999; 10: 354–65.

51. Fenton SSA, Schaubel DE, Desmeules M, et al. Hemodialysis versus peritoneal dialysis: A comparison of adjusted mortality rates. *Am J Kid Dis* 1997; 30: 334–42.

52. Collins AJ, Hao W, Xia H, et al. Mortality risks of peritoneal dialysis and hemodialysis. *Am J Kid Dis* 1999; 34: 1065–74.

53. Schaubel DE, Fenton SSA. Trends in mortality on peritoneal dialysis: Cnada, 1981–1997. *J Am Soc Nephrol* 2000; 11: 126–33.

54. Heaf JG, Lokkegaarg H, Madsen M. Initial survival advantage of peritoneal dialysis relative to hemodialysis. *Nephrol Dial Transplant* 2002; 17: 112–17.

55. Korevaar JC, Feith GW, Dekker FW, et al. Effect of starting with hemodialysis compared with peritoneal dialysis in patients new on dialysis treatment: A randomized controlled trial. *Kidney Int* 2003; 64: 2222–28.

56. Ganesh SK, Hulbert T, Port FK, et al. Mortality differences by dialysis modality among incident ESRD patients with and without coronary artery disease. *J Am Soc Nephrol* 2003; 14: 415–24.

57. Mehrotra R, Chiu Y-W, Kalantar-Zadeh K, Bargman J, Vonesh E. Similar outcomes with hemodialysis and peritoneal dialysis with similar outcomes for endstage renal disease treatment in United States [published online September 27, 2010]. *Arch Intern Med* doi: 10.1001/archinternmed.2010.352.

58. Davies S, Phillips L, Griffiths AM, et al. What really happens to people on long-term peritoneal dialysis? *Kidney Int* 1998; 54: 2207–17.

59. Kawaguchi Y, Hasegawa T, Nakayama M, et al. Issues affecting the longevity of continuous ambulatory peritoneal dialysis. *Kidney Int* 1997; 52 (suppl 62): S105–7.

60. Gokal R, Oreopoulos DG. Is long-term technique survival on CAPD possible? *Perit Dial Int* 1996; 16: 553–5.

61. Williams JD, Craig KJ, Ruhland CV, et al. The natural course of peritoneal membrane biology during peritoneal dialysis. *Kidney Int* 2003; 64 (suppl 88): S43–9.

62.   Dobbie JW, Anderson JD, Hind C. Long-term effects of peritoneal dialysis on peritoneal morphology. *Perit Dial Int* 1994; 14 (suppl 3): 16–20.

63.   Yanez-Mo M, Lara-Pezzi E, Selgas R, et al. Peritoneal dialysis and epithelial-to-mesenchymal transition of mesothelial cells. *N Eng J Med* 2003; 348: 403–13.

64.   Davies S, Bryan J, Phillips L, Russell GI. Longitudinal changes in peritoneal kinetics: The effect of peritoneal dialysis and peritonitis. *Nephrol Dial Transplant* 1996; 11: 498–506.

65.   Selgas R, Fernandes RMJ, Bosque E, et al. Functional longevity of the human peritoneum: How long is continuous peritoneal dialysis possible? Results of a prospective medium-term study. *Am J Kid Dis* 1994; 23: 64–73.

66.   Wang T, Hrimburger O, Waniewski J, et al. Increased peritoneal permeability is associated with decreased fluid and small solute removal and higher mortality in CAPD patients. *Nephrol Dial Transplant* 1998; 13: 1242–9.

67.   Churchill DN, Thorpe KE, Nolph KDA, et al. Increased peritoneal membrane transport is associated with decreased patient and technique survival for continuous peritoneal dialysis patients. *J Am Soc Nephrol* 1998; 9: 1285–92.

68.   Davies SJ, Phillips L, Russell GI. Peritoneal solute transport predicts survival on CAPD independently of residual renal function. *Nephrol Dial Transplant* 1998; 13: 962–8.

69.   Mactier RA, Sprosen TS, Gokal R, et al. Bicarbonate and bicarbonate/lactate peritoneal dialysis solutions for the treatment of infusion pain. *Kidney Int* 1998; 53: 1061–7.

70.   Topley N. In vitro biocompatibility of bicarbonate-based peritoneal dialysis solutions. *Perit Dial Int* 1997; 17: 42–7.

71.   Topley N, Coles GA, Williams JD. Biocompatibility studies on peritoneal cells. *Perit Dial Int* 1994; 14 (suppl 3): S21–8.

72.   Topley N, Kaur D, Petersen MM, et al. In vitro effects of bicarbonate and bicarbonate-lactate buffered peritoneal dialysis solutions on mesothelial and neutrophils function. *J Am Soc Nephrol* 1996; 7: 218–224.

73.   Yamamoto T, Sakakura T, Yamakawa M, et al. Clinical effects of long-term use of neutralized dialysate for continuous ambulatory peritoneal dialysis. *Nephron* 1992; 60: 324–9.

74.   Mak RH, DeFronzo RA. Glucose and insulin metabolism in uremia. *Nephron* 1992; 61: 377–382.

75.   Ramos JM, Heaton A, McGurk JG, et al. Sequential changes in serum lipids and their subfractions in patients receiving CAPD. *Nephron* 1983; 35: 20–23.

76.   De Vriese ASD, Mortier S, Lameire NH. What happens to the peritoneal membrane in long-term peritoneal dialysis. *Perit Dial Int* 2001; 21 (suppl 3): S9–18.

77.   Welten AGA, le Pool K, Ittersum FJV, et al. Biocompatibility of high versus low glucose regime on peritoneal cells of CAPD patients in a multi-centered study. *J Am Soc Nephrol* 2002; 13: 202A.

78.   Vardhan A, Zweers MM, Gokal R, Kreidet RT. A solutions portfolio approach in peritoneal dialysis. *Kidney Int* 2003; 64 (suppl 88): S114–123.

79.   Hoff CM. In vitro biocompatibility performance of physioneal. *Kidney Int* 2003; 64 (suppl 88): S57–74.

80. Wieslander A, Nordin MK, Kjellstrand PTT, Boberg UC. Toxicity of peritoneal dialysis fluids on cultured fibroblasts. *Kidney Int* 1991; 40: 77–79.

81. Witowski J, Wisniewska J, Korybalska K, et al. Prolonged exposure to glucose degradation products impairs viability and function of human peritoneal mesothelial cells. *J Am Soc Nephrol* 2001; 12: 2434–2441.

82. Witowski J, Jorres A, Koryblaska K, et al. Glucose degradation products in peritoneal dialysis fluids: Do they harm? *Kidney Int*, 2003; 63 (suppl 84): S148–51.

83. Witowski J, Jorres A, Koryblaska K, et al. Glucose degradation products in peritoneal dialysis fluids: Do they harm? *Kidney Int* 2003; 63 (suppl 84): S148–51.

84. Linden T, Cohen A, Deppisch R, et al. 3,4-Dideoxyglucosone-3-ene (3,4-DGE): a cytotoxic glucose degradation product in fluids for peritoneal dialysis. *Kidney Int* 2002; 62: 697–703.

85. Rippe B, Simonsen O, Heimburger O, et al. Long-term clinical effects of a peritoneal dialysis fluid with less glucose degradation products. *Kidney Int* 2001; 59: 348–57.

86. Ha H, Yu MR, Choi HN, et al. Effects of conventional and new peritoneal dialysis solutions on human peritoneal mesothelial cell viability and proliferation. *Perit Dial Int* 2000; 20 (suppl 5): S10–19.

87. Morgan LW, Wieslander A, Davies M, et al. Glucose degradation products (GDP) retard remesothelialization independently of D-glucose concentration. *Kidney Int* 2003; 64: 1854–66.

88. Miyata T, Devuyst O, Kurokawa K, Strihou CVYD. Towards better dialysis compatibility: Advances in the biochemistry and pathophysiology of the peritoneal membranes. *Kidney Int* 2002; 61: 375–86.

89. Maillard LC. Action des acides amines sur les sucres. Formation des melanoidines par voi methodique. *C R Acad Sci* 1912; I 154: 66–8.

90. Brownlee M, Cerami A, Vlassara H. Advanced glycosylation end products in tissue and the biochemical basis of diabetic complications. *N Engl J Med* 1988; 318: 1315–21.

91. Yamagishi S, Takeuchi M, Makita Z. Advanced glycation end products and the pathogenesis of diabetic nephropathy. *Contrib Nephrol* 2001; 134: 30–5.

92. Vlassara H, Palace MR. Diabetes and advanced glycation end products. *J Int Med* 2002; 251: 87–101.

93. Raj DSC, Choudhury D, Welbourne TC, Levi M. Advanced glycation end products: A nephrologist's perspective. *Am J Kidney Dis* 2000; 35: 365–80.

94. Nakamura S, Tachikawa T, Tobita K, et al. Role of advanced glycation end products and growth factors in peritoneal dysfunction. *Am J Kidney Dis* 2003; 41 (suppl 1): S61–67.

95. Nishida Y, Shao J, Kiribayashi K, et al. Advanced glycation end products reduce the viability of human peritoneal mesothelial cells. *Nephron* 1998; 80: 477–8.

96. Boulanger E, Wautier MP, Wutier JL, et al. AGEs bind to mesothelial cells via RAGE and stimulate VCAM-1 expression. *Kidney Int* 2002; 61: 148–56.

97. Wieslander A, Linden T, Kjellstrand P. Glucose degradation products in peritoneal dialysis fluids: How they can be avoided. *Perit Dial Int* 2001; 21 (suppl 3): S119–124.

98. Martis L, Henderson LW. Impact of terminal heat sterlization on the quality of peritoneal dialysis solutions. *Blood Purif* 1997; 15: 54–60.

99. Chung SH, Stenvinkel P, Bergstrom J, Lindholm B. Biocompatibility of new peritoneal dialysis solutions: What can we hope to achieve? *Perit Dial Int* 2000; 20 (suppl 5): S57–67.

100. Moberly JB, Mujais S, Gehr T, et al. Pharmacokinetics of icodextrin in peritoneal dialysis patients. *Kidney Int* 2002; 62 (suppl 81): S23–33.

101. Wolfson M, Ogrinc F, Mujais S. Review of clinical trial experience with icodextrin. *Kidney Int* 2002; 62 (suppl 81): S46–52.

102. Cooker LA, Holmes CJ, Hoff CM. Biocompatibility of icodextrin. *Kidney Int* 2002; 62 (suppl 81): S34–45.

103. Young GA, Kopple JD, Lindholm B, et al. Nutritional assessment of continuous ambulatory peritoneal dialysis. An international study. *Am J Kidney Dis* 1991; 17: 462–71.

104. Lopez EG, Lindholm B, Tranaeus A. Biocompatibility of new peritoneal dialysis solutions: Clinical experience. *Perit Dial Int* 2000; 20 (suppl 5): S48–56.

105. Lage C, Pischetsrieder M, Aufricht C, et al. First in vitro and in vivo experiences with staysafe balance, a pH-neural solution in a dual-chambered bag. *Perit Dial Int* 2000; 20 (suppl 5): S28–32.

106. Hoff CM. In vitro biocompatibility performance of physioneal. *Kidney Int* 2003; 64 (supp 88): S57–74.

107. Pecoits-Filho R, Tranaeus A, Lindholm B. Clinical trial experiences with physioneal. *Kidney Int* 2003; 64 (supp 88): S100–4.

108. Ayuzawa N, Ishibashi Y, Takazawa Y, Kume H, FujitaT. Peritoneal morphology after longterm peritoneal dialysis with biocompatible fluid: Recent clinical practice in Japan *Perit Dial Int* 2012; 32(2):159–167.

109. le Poole CY, Welten AGA, Weijmer MC, Valentijn RM, van Ittersum FJ, Wee PMT. Initiating CAPD with a regimen low in glucose and glucose degradation products, with icodextrin and amino acids (NEPP) is safe and efficacious. *Perit Dial Int* 2005; 25(S3):S64–S68.

110. le Poole CY, Welten AGA, Wee PMT, et al. A peritoneal dialysis regimen low in glucose and glucose degradation products results in increased cancer antigen 125 and peritoneal activation. *Perit Dial Int* 2011; doi: 10.3747/pdi.2010.00115.

111. le Poole CY, van Ittersum FJ, Valentijn RM, et al. NEPP peritoneal dialysis regimen has beneficial effects on plasma CEL and 3-DG, but not pentosidine, CML, and MGO *Perit Dial Int* 2012; 32: 45–54.

112. Miyata T, Kurokawa K, van Ypersele DSC. Advanced glycation and lipidoxidation end products: role of reactive carbonyl compounds generated during carbohydrate and lipid metabolism. *J Am Soc Nephrol* 2000; 11: 1744-52.

113. Hobbs AJ, Higgs A, Noncada S. Inhibition of nitric oxide synthase as a potential therapeutic target. *Ann Rev Pharmacol Toxicol* 1999; 39: 191-220.

114. De Vriese AS, Tilton RG, Seephan CC, Lameire N. Diabetes-induced microvascular proliferation and hyperpermeability in the peritoneum: role of vascular endothelial growth factor. *J Am Soc Nephrol* 2001; 12: 1734-41.

PRESCRIBING PERITONEAL DIALYSIS

J. BARGMAN, R. SAXENA

Although PD is decidedly more "low tech" compared to HD, the dialysis prescription takes more thought and planning in its execution. Whereas HD machines and filters are manufactured to exacting standards so that the membrane characteristics are predictable in each dialysis treatment, from day to day, transport properties of the peritoneal membrane are variable from patient to patient, and even within the same patient over time.

This chapter will review how to characterize the transport properties of the peritoneal membrane with the Peritoneal Equilibration Test (PET); and how to prescribe PD with special reference to solute transport, UF, minimizing complications, and optimizing convenience and adherence to therapy by the patient.

THE PERITONEAL EQUILIBRATION TEST

The purpose of the PET is to quantitate the solute transport properties and UF capacity of the peritoneal membrane. These characteristics will be unique to the patient, and may change over time (1).

This test is easily performed by the PD nurse. It is recommended that the PET be performed at least 1 month after insertion of the PD catheter. The catheter insertion procedure, by necessity, disrupts the local environment of the peritoneum and its function during recovery may not be reflective of the function of the membrane once the patient is established on PD. Furthermore, if the patient is commencing PD with residual kidney function, the dose of PD is not all that crucial, as discussed later in this chapter, and the PET does not have to be used to design the prescription.

The baseline PET is usually performed about 2 to 3 months after the start of therapy.

The test involves the instillation of 2 liters of 2.5% or 4.25% dextrose dialysis fluid into the drained peritoneal cavity. The patient is instructed to roll from one side to the other to facilitate good distribution and admixture of fluid with whatever unintended residual volume is left from the last drain. Samples of dialysis fluid are collected at baseline, 2 hours, and 4 hours after instillation. The samples are analyzed for glucose, urea, and creatinine levels. Some analysis units also measure sodium concentration in the dialysis fluid. A blood test at the midpoint (2 hours) is drawn for creatinine, urea, and sometimes sodium.

The PET was originally described using 2.5% dextrose solution. However, using the 4.25% solution will maximize the osmotic pressure and provide the best stimulus for UF. Some workers feel that the 4.25% solution is a better test of peritoneal membrane function, and that it does not materially affect the solute transport values. Currently some units use 2.5% and others 4.25% for the PET (2).

During the 4-hour test period, urea and creatinine will diffuse from the blood into the dialysate. At the same time, glucose will diffuse along its own concentration gradient from the dialysis fluid into the blood. Just how quickly these small solutes cross the peritoneal membrane is measured by the PET. The dialysis-to-plasma ratio (D/P) of creatinine or urea will be higher if these solutes move quickly across the membrane. For example, urea is small and easily diffusible. Therefore, after a 4-hour dwell, the concentration of urea in the dialysate will approach the same concentration in the blood. Hence, the D/P urea will be close to 1. For this reason, urea is not a good discriminator of trans-peritoneal transport. Creatinine, on the other hand, is a larger and more slow-moving solute and discriminates better across transport types. In a rapid transporter, after a 4-hour dwell, the concentration of creatinine in the dialysate sample is typically at least 80% of the creatinine concentration in the blood sample. It has been determined, empirically, that patients on PD can be categorized into quartiles of transport based on the D/P creatinine: rapid, rapid-average, slow-average, and slow (1).

Table 8.1. Classification of Transport Characteristics

Category	Transport Character Ultrafiltration (in ml)	D/P Creatinine ratio at 4 hours
Rapid	(270)–35	0.82–1.03
Rapid-Average	35–320	0.65–0.81
Slow-Average	320–600	0.50–0.64
Slow	600–1276	0.34–0.49

Peritoneal membrane transport characteristics are classified into 4 categories, based upon the D/P creatinine ratio at 4 hours.

We cannot measure D/P glucose because the glucose diffusing out of the peritoneal cavity is almost instantly metabolized. Therefore the plasma glucose does not rise in concert with the fall in dialysate glucose. For this reason, the flux of glucose out of the peritoneal cavity is measured by calculating the difference between the concentration of glucose remaining in the peritoneal cavity at the end of the 4-hour dwell to how much was instilled at time zero. This metric is the D4/D0 glucose. A rapid transporter will have less glucose remaining, so the D4/D0 will be a lower number than achieved by a slower transporter. The PET form provides a place to record both creatinine and glucose flux, but in reality most people use the D/P creatinine in judging the transport status of the patient.

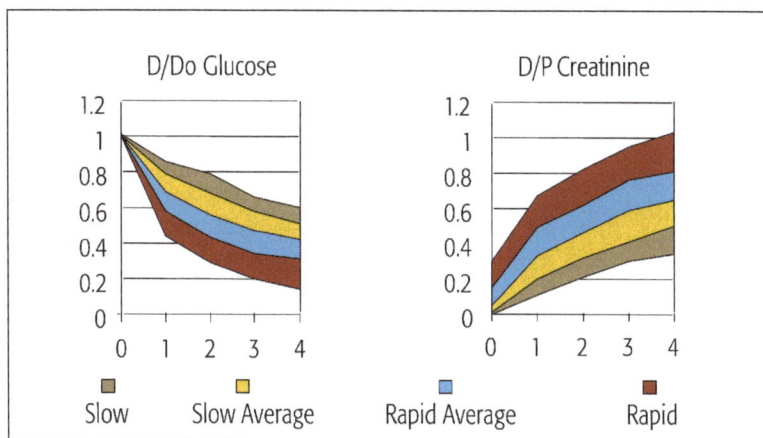

D/Do Glucose   **D/P Creatinine**

Slow   Slow Average   Rapid Average   Rapid

Figure 8.1. The glucose dialysate to dialysate ratio at time zero (D/D0) and dialysate to plasma ratios (D/P) of creatinine at various dwell times during the standard peritoneal equilibration test.

Peritoneal Equilibration Test and the Implication for Ultrafiltration

The faster the glucose diffuses out of the peritoneal cavity, the faster the osmotic gradient, which is responsible for UF, will dissipate. Therefore, rapid transporters will have limited UF with dextrose-based dialysis solutions, while slow transporters will maintain their osmotic gradient longer and have better UF. Because the slow transporters will have more convective removal of solutes because of the UF, their total (diffusive and convective) solute removal may not be all that different from that seen with rapid transporters, where small solute diffusive clearance is high but convective clearance low (because of less UF). That is why "high" and "low" transporters may be misnomers, and "rapid" and "slow" is preferred.

Rapid transporters will achieve better UF with shorter dwell times. If the patient elects to dialyse via cycler, the overnight dwells can quite easily be short. For example, 4 exchanges over 8 hours will allow for no more than a 90 minute dwell (there is obligatory time lost for inflow and outflow). This dwell time is short enough that even rapid transporters will maintain an osmotic gradient and be able to remove fluid. However, the problem is the long day dwell, which, in this example, will be 16 hours (24 minus 8). If a single dextrose-based day dwell is used, there will be significant absorption of solutes, sodium, and water so that any net fluid loss achieved by UF overnight may be totally negated by absorption during this long day dwell.

To minimize absorption during the long day dwell, icodextrin can be used instead of a hypertonic dextrose-based dialysis solution. The UF that occurs by colloid osmosis with icodextrin occurs slowly and can continue for 14–16 hours in many, but not all, patients (3). If icodextrin is unavailable or not practical, the patient can be left dry during the day so that there is no risk of net fluid absorption. However, if the patient has lost residual kidney function, the loss of all these hours of dialysis can lead to under dialysis and uremia. While there are no studies that have examined this rigorously, day dry should not be considered unless the patient has at least 5 ml/min residual GFR or the patient is palliative. Some compromise prescriptions have the patient carry fluid for part of the day and stay dry for several hours.

The rapid transporter who elects to perform CAPD will face the same problem of absorption during the nighttime long dwell. In this case, however, the long dwell is usually about 8 hours instead of 15 or 16 with APD. Again, if there is sufficient residual GFR, the patient on CAPD can be dry overnight, or else use a hypertonic dextrose solution or icodextrin for the overnight dwell.

Importantly, if the patient has sizable residual kidney function, even if they absorb dialysate with the long dwell, they may remain euvolemic because of renal salt and water excretion. In that case, no adjustment necessarily has to be made to the prescription, but residual kidney function must be monitored closely because of the risk of onset of fluid overload with diminishing urine output.

Finally, it is important to consider the use of loop diuretics or metolazone to augment renal salt and water excretion (4). Diuretics and dietary salt restriction are adjunctive measures to help maintain euvolemia in the dialysis patient.

Peritoneal Equilibration Test and Solute Transport

Rapid transporters will experience fast solute removal that is threatened only by back-absorption of dialysate during the long dwell. On the other hand, slow transporters require longer dwell times to allow for trans-membrane flux of solutes. Frequent short exchanges are counterproductive for slow transporters because the dialysis fluid will not dwell long enough for solute equilibration and is further compromised by the lost time of inflow and outflow. Because of this, some have advised that slow transporters should not undertake cycler dialysis. However, the decision about APD versus CAPD should not usually be contingent on transport status, but more for lifestyle considerations (see below). If a slow transporter wants to undertake APD, they should conduct night cycling as long as is convenient for them, and then not have more than three exchanges. For example, three exchanges over ten hours should allow for a reasonable length of dwell. If the patient has a mid-day exchange, the regimen is then quite similar to CAPD, but with the day and night exchanges reversed.

Solute Transport and "Adequate" Dialysis

It is unclear how much dialysis is needed to maintain patients in their best state of health. Randomized, controlled studies of dose of dialysis, as quantitated by small solute kinetics (weekly Kt/V_{urea} or creatinine clearance) have been unable to show an association of dose with survival. (5,6) There are many confounding issues to dose and survival, including the following:

- the contribution of residual kidney function
- the variability among patients
- the neglect of the role of "middle molecules" and their contribution to patient well-being and survival

Many national renal organizations have put forward recommendations for dose of PD. Some more "generous" targets have been proposed so those wanting to prescribe more, rather than the minimum, amount of dialysis would not be censured for doing so. This lead to the unexpected consequence of a small solute target being misinterpreted as a minimum prescription— with the result that many patients on PD were undertaking onerous amounts of exchanges every day. Currently most renal organizations who are undertaking guidelines are settling on a minimum total (renal + peritoneal) weekly Kt/V_{urea} of 1.7 (7). Given the negative outcome studies mentioned above, there is now less emphasis on small solute targets, although many large dialysis chains unfortunately are still focused on these.

PRESCRIPTIONS TO MINIMIZE COMPLICATIONS

The infusion of 2 liters or more of dialysis fluid into the peritoneal cavity leads to an increase in intra-abdominal pressure (IAP) (8). This pressure rise can be mitigated somewhat by limiting the volume infused or by assuming the supine posture. However, activities such as exercise, straining at stool, and vigorous coughing can lead to very high IAP when there is dialysis fluid in situ. Complications of IAP include hernias and leak of dialysis fluid out of the peritoneal cavity. The fluid can leak into the soft tissues of the abdominal wall through a rent in the supporting soft tissues, or a breach in the peritoneal cavity because of a hernia itself. Fluid can leak across defects in the hemi diaphragm (usually on the right side) and gather in the pleural space, a complication referred to as PD hydrothorax. If the processus vaginalis, which connects the peritoneal cavity to the tunica vaginalis in the scrotum or labia, has not undergone normal obliteration in fetal life, dialysis fluid can travel from the cavity to the scrotum or labia, leading to hydrocele or labial edema.

Patients at risk for complications of PD as a result of raised IAP include those who are obese, elderly, malnourished, or those on long-term corticosteroid therapy or mTor inhibitors such as rapamycin. A group of patients at special risk for hernias and leaks are those with polycystic kidney disease. Not only do massively enlarged kidneys protrude into the peritoneal space reducing the volume available for dialysis fluid, but these patients also have a connective tissue defect that predisposes them to hernia and leak even without very enlarged kidneys.(9)

In the patient at risk for complications related to increased IAP, some thought has to be put into the prescription. Two major factors that raise the IAP are the volume of dialysate (including UF) and the position of the patient. An ideal prescription for the at-risk patient would entail night cycler dialysis, wherein the patient is supine for the procedure. If there is sufficient residual kidney function, the patient could remain dry during the day when IAP is higher. If a day dwell is needed, it could be a smaller volume, such as a 1-liter fill coming off the cycler, and a 1-liter mid-day exchange. If the at-risk patient is on CAPD, more frequent day dwells of smaller volumes could be used, and the larger volume used overnight.

Any patient on PD should be warned about activities that can increase the IAP. We usually ask that their job entail no heavy lifting, such as anything more than 10 pounds. They should be instructed to drain their fluid before taking part in activities that could increase the pressure, such as aerobics classes or weightlifting.

PRESCRIPTIONS TO OPTIMIZE CONVENIENCE AND ADHERENCE TO THERAPY

Since PD is a home-based therapy, adherence to the treatment is never certain. There are computer cards that can be inserted into the cyclers that track the treatment, and the amount of dialysis fluid ordered from the supplier can also be monitored. Younger patients have a higher rate of non-adherence to the dialysis prescription, which is perhaps not surprising given the rigidity and regimentation of the prescription. Furthermore, it is my impression that the kind of patient who chooses to do home therapy in the first place also, frequently, wants to be autonomous in carrying it out.

Those looking after home patients have to be aware of this uncertainty and adopt a degree of flexibility in the dialysis prescription. Within the confines of prescribing adequate dialysis to keep the patient well, the prescription should be tailored to the lifestyle of the patient, and not the other way around.

Patients should be educated about the differences between CAPD and APD, and in most cases should be able to choose the therapy that best suits them. For example, a patient with frequent nocturia may be reluctant to undertake night cycler, given the many trips to the toilet that occur for that patient. It is important to discuss with the patient how he/she spends their day and their night. Are they restless sleepers who frequently get out of bed to watch television or have a sandwich? What time do they usually get out of bed in the morning and go to bed at night? Prescribing a 9-hour night-cycling regimen will be onerous for the patient who sleeps no more than 6 hours. A "mid-day" exchange does not have to be exactly in the middle of the day. If the patient works in an office it may be easy to do an exchange at lunch, but the same cannot be said for the patient who works as a crossing guard. For some it will be more convenient to do the "mid-day" exchange after coming home from work or from school.

If the patient has residual kidney function, it may be helpful to use it in the adequacy calculations and prescribe less PD. Examples of incremental PD in the face of residual kidney function include CAPD for 2–3 exchanges daily, or night cycles and day dry, or 2–3 exchanges overnight with a long dwell during the day that may or may not be drained out at dinnertime to avoid absorption. Again, these prescriptions should be agreed upon in consultation with the patient. The patient should be allowed to miss exchanges or even a day of dialysis for special occasions. If the patient is prescribed incremental dialysis, the residual kidney function must be monitored routinely and the patient warned that the dose of dialysis will be increased when there is evidence of decline in the kidney function.

SMALL SOLUTE CLEARANCE OR Kt/V$_{urea}$

Another tool used to assess PD is small solute clearance or Kt/V$_{urea}$. Urea clearance is conventionally used as a surrogate for small solute clearance. A large prospective study comprising patients for Canadian and USA PD centers (CANUSA study), observed that higher small solute clearance would improve patient survival (10). Consequently, the National Kidney Foundation's K/DOQI recommended a weekly total solute removal in terms of Kt/V$_{urea}$ for CAPD of 2.0 or more per week. Higher targets were chosen for continuous cycling PD (CCPD) and patients on nocturnal intermittent peritoneal dialysis (NIPD). A more recent randomized study, the Adequacy of PD in Mexico Study, comparing 2 levels of PD prescription, showed that patients with lower Kt/V$_{urea}$ had similar survival as those with higher Kt/V$_{urea}$ (5). This suggests no benefit on survival for greater small-molecule peritoneal clearance. This was further suggested by another randomized trial of CAPD patients from Hong Kong comparing 3 levels of total Kt/V_{urea}, with the lowest group randomized to a total Kt/V_{urea} of 1.5 to 1.7, with no difference in survival (6). As a result, K/DOQI reduced the recommended goal for Kt/V_{urea} to 1.7 in the revised guidelines for patients on CAPD (11).

Kt/V_{urea} is calculated as weekly urea clearance normalized to total body water which is approximately the volume of distribution of urea. Thus **K** is the urea clearance, **t** is time in days and **V** is the total body water. The anthropometric formulas such as Watson or Humes are used to estimate total body water (**V**) (12,13). However, by using actual body weight, these formulas may overestimate body water in obese patients on PD (14). Furthermore, they underestimate body water in patients with volume expansion on PD and overestimate body water in those with volume deficit (14). Given that **V** represents the volume of distribution of urea, only the weight of tissues in which urea diffuses should be used for this calculation. Therefore, patient's ideal or standard body weight (rather than actual weight) should be considered in the calculation of **V**.

Dialysate and residual renal Kt/V_{urea} are calculated separately and added together to compute total Kt/V_{urea}.

Dialysate **K** is calculated by multiplying the total dialysate volume in 24 hours by the ratio of dialysate and plasma urea, that is: total effluent volume in 24 hours × D/P urea.

Residual renal **K** is calculated by multiplying the total urine volume in 24 hours by the ratio of urine and plasma urea, that is: total urine volume in 24 hours × U/P urea.

Thus, total Kt/V_{urea} is the sum of the weekly dialysate Kt/V_{urea} plus the weekly renal Kt/V_{urea}.

Weekly Dialysate (PD) Kt/Vurea =

{[24-hr Drain Volume × (Dialysate Urea / Plasma Urea)] × 7 days} / Volume of Distribution of Urea

Weekly Renal Kt/Vurea =

{[24-hr Urine Volume × (Urin Urea / Plasma Urea)] × 7 days} / Volume of Distribution of Urea

Total Kt/Vurea =

Weekly Dialysate (Peritoneal) Kt/Vurea + Weekly Renal Kt/Vurea

For Example:

For example, a 70-year-old male on CAPD doing 4 exchanges of 2L has 2125 cc of total UF in 24 hours, has serum urea nitrogen (BUN) of 14.1 mg/dl, and dialysate urea nitrogen of 12.7 mg/dl. He weighs 53 kg. Thus, the total drain volume is 4×2000 cc + 2125 cc = 10,125 cc. The volume of distribution of urea is equal to total body water, which is approximately $0.6 \times$ the patient's weight, in this case 53 kg, for a total of 31.8 L or 31,800 cc.

Thus, weekly Kt/V_{urea} is:

$$\{ [10,125 \times (12.7 / 14.1)] \times 7 \} / 31,800 = 2.01$$

So what does Kt/V_{urea} = 2.01 signify?

Kt/V_{urea} is a number with no units or dimensions. It is not a measure of dialysis adequacy. It does not indicate good or poor clearance. It is a measure of dialysis dose. Kt/V_{urea} of 2.01 simply means that 2.01 volumes of distribution of urea are completely cleared of urea in 1 week. Whether this amount of clearance is adequate or not will depend upon patient's symptoms, nutrition, and volume status. Therefore, apart from routinely checking Kt/V_{urea}, it is of paramount importance in routine assessment of patients on PD to also monitor RRF, evaluate volume status and blood pressure control, assess nutritional status, and ensure absence of uremic symptoms.

REFERENCES

1. Twardowski Z, Nolph K, Khanna R, et al. Peritoneal equilibration test. *Perit Dial Bull* 1987; 7: 138–47.

2. Pride E, Gustafson J, Graham A, et al. Comparison of a 2.5% and a 4.25% dextrose peritoneal equilibration test. *Perit Dial Int* 2002; 2: 365–70.

3. Mistry C. The beginning of icodextrin. *Perit Dial Int* 2011; 11 Suppl 2: S49–52.

4. Medcalf J, Harris K, Walls J. Role of diuretics in the preservation of residual renal function in patients on continuous ambulatory peritoneal dialysis. *Kidney Int* 2001; 59(3): 1128–33.

5. Paniagua R, Amato D, Vonesh E, et al. Effect of increased peritoneal clearances on mortality rates in peritoneal dialysis: ADEMEX, a prospective, randomized controlled trial. *J Am Soc Nephrol* 2002; 13(5): 1307–20.

6. Lo WK, Ho Y, Li K, et al. Effect of Kt/V on survival and clinical outcome in CAPD patients in a randomized prospective study. *Kidney Int* 2003; 64(2): 649–56.

7. Lo WK, Bargman J, Burkart J, et al. Guideline on targets for solute and fluid removal in adult patients on chronic peritoneal dialysis. *Perit Dial Int* 2006; 26(2): 191–7.

8. Twardowski Z, Khanna R, Nolph K, et al. Intraabdominal pressures during natural activities in patients treated with continuous ambulatory peritoneal dialysis. *Nephron* 1986; 44(2): 129–35.

9.   Li L, Szeto CC, Kwan B, et al. Peritoneal dialysis as the first-line renal replacement therapy in patients with autosomal dominant polycystic kidney disease. *Am J Kidney Dis* 2011; 57(6): 903–7.

10. The CANUSA Peritoneal Dialysis Study Group. Adequacy of dialysis and nutrition in continuous peritoneal dialysis: association with clinical outcomes. *J Am Soc Nephrol* 1996; 7(2): 198–207.

11. Peritoneal Dialysis Work Group 2006. Clinical practice guidelines for peritoneal dialysis adequacy, update 2006; pp 117–225 National Kidney Foundation, 2006.

12. Watson PE, Watson ID, Batt RD. Total body water volumes for adult males and females estimated from simple anthropometric measurements. *Am J Clin Nutr* 1980; 33: 27–39.

13. Hume R, Weyers E. Relationship between total body water and surface area in normal and obese subjects. *J Clin Pathol* 1971; 24: 234–238.

14. Johansson AC, Samuelsson O, Attman PO, et al. Limitations in anthropometric calculations of total body water in patients on peritoneal dialysis. *J Am Soc Nephrol* 2001; 12:568–573.

COMMENTS ON PLACING PERITONEAL CATHETERS IN CHILDREN

M. BRANDT

Peritoneal dialysis is used more commonly than vascular access in children with ESRD but is often more challenging than placing catheters in adults. The technical challenge of placing catheters in children is compounded by the dramatic differences in the size of pediatric patients. Successful catheter placement requires careful planning and technical expertise (1).

There are a limited number of catheters manufactured for children; therefore finding the "ideal" catheter is often problematic. Catheter length, which is listed by the manufacturer, refers to the total length (tip to tip when straightened and uncoiled). The more important length for the surgeon is the distance from the first (peritoneal) cuff to the tip of the intra-abdominal segment. Although there are no conclusive data, most surgeons and nephrologists feel that catheters with coiled intra-abdominal segments have less occlusion. Swan Neck catheters may allow for better orientation of the exit site, but they are more difficult to place in children with thin abdominal walls. In very small children, single cuff catheters are preferred since it is difficult to position the second (subcutaneous) cuff.

Children do not come in 1 size; nor should PD catheters. Their needs, physiques, and capabilities require different catheter styles and sizes. In choosing the best available PD catheter for an individual child, the following conditions should be met.

1. The catheter should be the appropriate length to allow placement into the most dependent portion of the pelvis, without creating an unnatural bend or kink in the catheter.
2. The cuff, if single, should be extra-peritoneal and firmly anchored in fascia.
3. If a second cuff is present, it should be positioned 1.5–2.0 cm from the exit site.
4. The exit site should be away from the diaper or belt line and directed in a lateral or, preferably, downward direction.

Peritoneal dialysis catheter systems are designed in various configurations to meet the specific needs of infant, pediatric, and adolescent patients. Pediatric catheters are available in multiple sizes and styles and in cuff options appropriate to the child's specific physique and needs (acute and chronic).

SURGICAL TECHNIQUE

The incision for placing a PD catheter is chosen to minimize the total number of incisions the child will need over a lifetime of dialysis. In general, a midline skin incision is used (Figure 9.1). In some children, a periumbilical incision may provide access as well. Like adults, the midline fascia should not be used to enter the abdomen. A vertical incision is made in the anterior fascia of the rectus muscle, and the muscle fibers spread (but not cut) to expose the posterior rectus sheath. If an omentectomy is performed, a vertical incision is made in the posterior fascia as well. If no omentectomy is needed, a purse-string suture is placed around the peritoneal incision (including the posterior rectus fascia) and later tied snugly around the PD catheter. Many surgeons will place a laparoscopic trocar through the incisions to inspect the inguinal rings. Inguinal hernias are common in children and can be repaired when the catheter is placed, if they are identified. A stylet is inserted into the catheter in order to guide the catheter through the posterior rectus sheath incision into the dependent pelvis. It is preferable to place the catheter tip slightly lateral to the midline to avoid compression from the rectum or bladder.

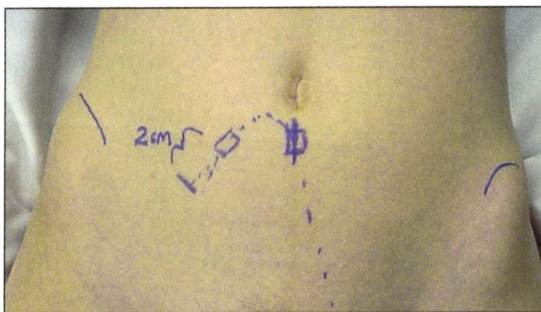

Figure 9.1. Planning Catheter Placement
Note the small midline incision, the 2 cm distance from the subcutaneous cuff to the exit site, and the downward facing exit site.

The next step is to fix the peritoneal cuff between the posterior and anterior rectus sheath. The previously placed purse string is tied snugly around the catheter and the needle used to attach the cuff to the anterior surface of the posterior sheath. A small incision is made lateral to the vertical incision in the anterior sheath and the catheter is tunneled obliquely to the lateral incision (Figure 9.2). For single-cuff catheters, the lateral incision in the anterior sheath should be as small as possible. If a subcutaneous cuff is tunneled through the rectus muscle, this opening may become large enough to require a second purse string. The catheter is then tunneled laterally out the anterior fascia. It is very important that this fascial opening be kept small so that the catheter fits tightly through it.

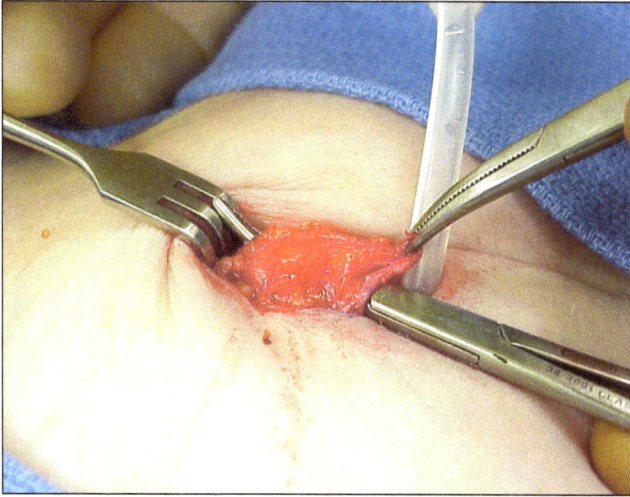

Figure 9.2. Lateral Incision in the Rectus Sheath
A hemostat is used to make a lateral incision through the rectus muscle. The catheter will be inserted under the sheath and through the incision.

The exit site is chosen in order to a) insure that the catheter points laterally or inferiorly, b) allow placement of the subcutaneous cuff 1.5 to 2.0 centimeters from the exit site, and c) avoid the area of the diaper and/or gastrostomy feeding tube (Figure 9.1). It is not uncommon to have to place the exit site in unorthodox positions to achieve these goals, for example, a presternal site. The exit site should be as small as possible to avoid catheter movement; it should be relatively difficult to pull the catheter through it. Excising a small circle of skin, rather than a linear incision, may allow a tighter fit. This can be accomplished with a skin biopsy puncture as described in Chapter 2 (Figure 2.34–2.38). Although the ideal is to place the exit site so the catheter exits in a downward direction, this is only completely possible in children if a Swan Neck catheter is being used. Bending a straight catheter into a position to achieve a downward pointing exit site will often create too much torque, which can result in intraperitoneal displacement of the catheter or cuff extrusion (Figure 9.3). (This is not the case in adults where a larger abdominal cavity allows for a wider bend with minimal resistance from the catheter's shape memory.) A hemostat or large "tunneler" must not be used to tunnel the catheter since it will dilate the tract. A metal "pin" with a hole drilled in 1 end (such as a Steinman pin) can be used instead. The catheter can be sutured to the end of the pin, which is then used to pull the catheter through the subcutaneous tissue. Again, the size of the exit site should be so small that some force is required to pull the catheter through it, creating a snug fit between the catheter and the skin.

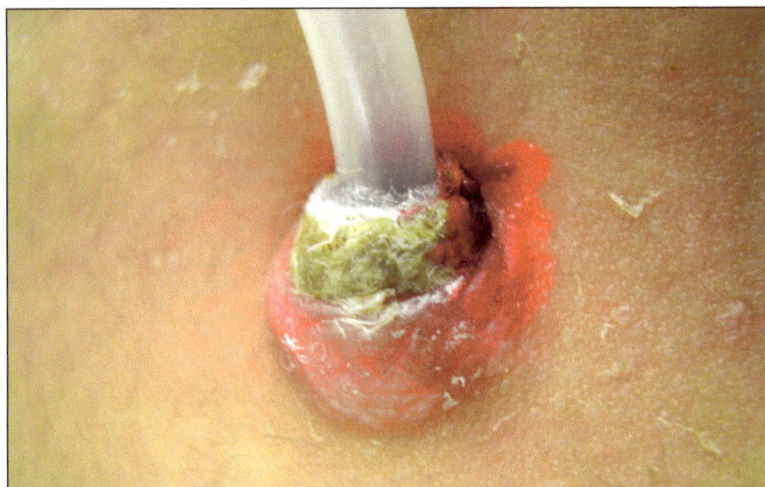

Figure 9.3. Cuff Extruding through the Skin
Cuff extrusion through the skin is a devastating complication and an indication of poor surgical technique related to exit site creation and cuff location.

A child with prune belly syndrome and poor development of the abdominal muscles, causing wrinkled skin, may present anatomical difficulties when placing a PD catheter (Figure 9.4).

The catheter is then tested while the patient is still under anesthesia. Saline with heparin (10 unit/cc) is instilled into the peritoneal cavity and allowed to flow out of the catheter by gravity (siphon). If there is not a steady, free flow at this point, the catheter must be revised. If necessary, the abdomen can be insufflated via the catheter and a 3 mm port placed to introduce a camera. Also, in most children, a less invasive 3 mm laparoscopic instrument can be inserted through the abdominal wall, remote from the PD catheter incisions, without an extra port in place, if the catheter needs to be repositioned.

No sutures should be placed at the exit site as this increases the risk of granulation tissue and exit-site infection. However, it is important to secure the catheter using a fixation device (such as a Foley catheter fixation or a device from interventional radiology).

Dressing the PD catheter and wounds involves several important steps, similar to that in an adult, but often requires modification according to special circumstances, including the size of the child. Suggested dressing material is pictured in Figure 2.48. Benzoin or Mastisol Adhesive Liquid helps to place the adhesive sterile closure strip on the incisions. A folded, incised gauze placed around the catheter at the exit site, keeps the exit site dry and eliminates catheter contact with the skin. A second layer of gauze on top of the Steri-Strip and the incised gauze will prevent the catheter and clamp from coming in contact with the skin. One or two adhesive film dressings are placed over this gauze. The rolled up catheter is then placed on top of the transparent film, making sure no catheter part or clamp is in contact with the skin. A layer of gauze is placed over the rolled up catheter to facilitate removal and dressing changes, as at no point should the adhesive dressing stick to the catheter or its parts. Place 2–3 adhesive film dressings over this gauze, taking care to avoid adhering the film to the catheter (Figure 2.54). One or two more transparent film dressings may be needed for a complete seal. The dressing is left in place for 7–10 days, although it must be changed if it becomes loose or soiled.

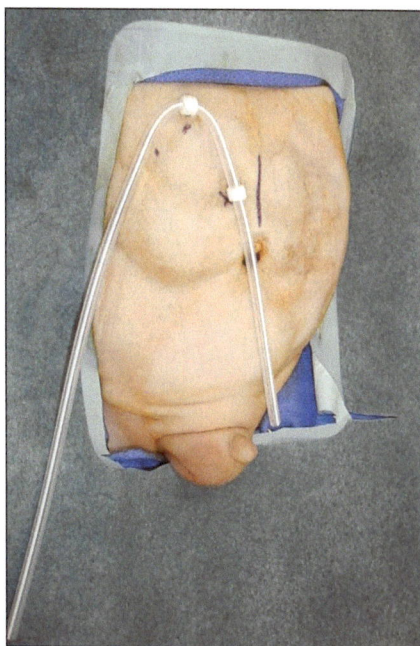

Figure 9.4. Prune Belly Syndrome in a Child
A child with prune belly syndrome involving poor development of the abdominal muscles and wrinkled skin may present anatomical difficulties when placing a PD catheter.

REFERENCE

Brandt ML, Brewer ED. *Peritoneal Dialysis. In Dialysis Therapy.* 5th ed. Philadelphia, PA: Hanley & Belfus, Inc.; 2007.

MANAGEMENT OF
PERITONEAL DIALYSIS COMPLICATIONS

I. DAVIDSON, R. SAXENA, M. YOO

Despite recent advances in peritoneal catheter technology and implantation techniques, catheter related complications lead to significant morbidity and treatment failure in up to 20% of patients on PD. The catheter related complications are classified as infectious and non-infectious, and can occur early (within 2 months of implantation), implicating surgical technique; or late (beyond 2 months), indicating catheter and PD exchange treatment issues.

COMPLICATIONS

Catheter related complications—leaks, peritonitis, obstruction, or hernias—may occur in up to 70% of cases over the lifetime of the PD catheter (1). The following text summarizes the most common complications related to PD. The more unusual PD complications are mentioned in this chapter, and covered in greater depth in Volume IV: Dialysis Access Case Reports. The case reports include "simulated' cases combining several unusual dialysis problems for maximal teaching impact.

Non-infectious Complications

Hernias
A variety of hernias have been described in patients on PD including incisional (the most common), inguinal, and umbilical, as well as hernias associated with the catheter placement site. Hernias are commonly related to long-term PD use. A cumulative incidence of 5–15% has been reported (2). They are more common when the incision is made at the midline. Hernias may first become apparent following implantation of the catheter due to increased IAP related to the volume of dialysate instilled. The position of the patient (supine position generates the lowest IAP for a given volume of intraperitoneal fluid compared to the sitting or upright position) and events such as coughing and straining can predispose hernia development, particularly in patients with congenital or acquired weakness or defects in the abdomen. Other risk factors include malnutrition, immunosuppressant drugs, several pregnancies, and a weak anterior abdominal wall. Development of hernias is not associated with body surface area, PD modality, volume of dialysate instilled, time of

largest dwell, or type of catheter used (3). Individuals with polycystic kidney disease while on PD have an increased risk for hernia development, possibly related to IAP or a connective tissue defect (4,5).

Hernias may present as a painless bulge, which is easily reducible. The presence of pain suggests an incarcerated or strangulated loop of bowel and indicates a serious complication, most commonly seen with umbilical hernias. A small hernia diagnosed before surgery can be repaired at the time of PD catheter placement. Symptomatic hernias occurring after initiation of PD should also be repaired. Peritoneal dialysis can often be resumed postoperatively by using low-volume exchanges (4–5 exchanges of 1–2 L) in a supine position (ideally with a nighttime cycler) for 2–4 weeks. Conversion to HD is not necessary and is not recommended in most instances.

Catheter Leakage

Up to 5% of patients undergoing PD may experience dialysate leaks (6) from an opening or a tear in the peritoneal membrane. Leaks can occur at any time after placement of a PD catheter. The risk factors for the development of leaks include poor surgical technique (such as a midline instead of a paramedian incision, and imprecise closure of the rectus fascia), a weak abdominal wall from multiple previous operations, multiple pregnancies, obesity, polycystic kidney disease, steroid use, and increased abdominal-wall tension (brought on by events such as high dialysate volume, constipation, coughing, severe straining, and lifting heavy weights). Age, sex, weight, catheter type, or particular insertion method do not seem to be associated with leaks (6). Initiating PD exchanges immediately after surgery and the use of a midline surgical approach are particularly associated with a higher risk of early leaks.

Early (<2 months) external leaks at the exit site or incision site are often related to poor surgical technique—most commonly, imprecise closure of the rectus fascia. Early surgical-site leaks are obvious and apparent soon after the initiation of PD exchanges. A "watertight" purse-string suture around the catheter as it exits the peritoneum, and a secure peritoneal cuff are key in preventing surgical-site leaks. See Chapters 2 and 4 for detailed surgical techniques. For best results, allow 3 to 4 weeks for healing to take place before initiation of fluid exchanges. Schedule the initial exchanges in gradually increasing volumes and administer them with the patient resting horizontally.

Late (> 2months) internal leaks into the abdominal wall, genitalia, or pleural cavity are related to a mechanical tear or a genetic defect in the peritoneal membrane (7). Symptoms of late leaks are subtle and include drainage around the catheter; subcutaneous swelling or edema of the abdominal wall; weight gain, genital edema; and reduced dialysate effluent volumes, often mistaken for ultra-filtration failure (6). Late leaks tend to develop during the first year of PD, and are rare beyond the third year (6).

Internal leaks are difficult to diagnose. Imaging techniques such as plain abdominal radiography or computed tomography (CT) (8,9) with intraperitoneal radio-contrast solution injected into the PD catheter; or intraperitoneal infusion of a radioisotope (technetium-tagged albumin) followed by peritoneal scintigraphy (10) may be useful. The most common approach to determine the exact site of the leakage is with a CT after infusion of 2 L of dialysis fluid mixed with a radio-contrast material (6).

Treatment includes surgical repair, with temporary transfer to HD or attempted low-volume nocturnal PD with a cycler. Most early leaks respond favorably to a temporary halt of fluid exchanges for a period of 2–3 weeks to allow small peritoneal defects to seal. Four to five low-volume exchanges (1000–1500 cc per exchange) with a nighttime cycler for 2–4 weeks, is often effective in treating early leaks, particularly when some RRF (GFR=5–10 cc/min) is present. Late leaks, weeks after placement of the PD catheter, as well as large early leaks, are unlikely to close with conservative management alone. Surgical repair is often needed in these situations. Successful use of fibrin glue to control catheter leaks (after failure to recover with conservative therapy) has been reported (11). Repair of a large defect is difficult and tends to lead to other even more serious complications, such as infections in particular. Removing and placing a new catheter (after a 3–4 week recovery) at a new site often presents the only safe option. A large leak in the presence of infection warrants removal of the catheter. Older catheters that have been in place for an extended period of time can also present with a large leak due to mechanical failure (i.e. fracture) of the catheter itself. Depending on the distance from the skin exit-site, catheter fractures can be repaired with prepackaged commercial patch kits under antibiotic treatment. Clinical judgment will determine the best action to follow, taking into consideration the patient's medical risk and healing progress since catheter placement, and the other dialysis options available to the patient. The experience of the center's team must also be taken into consideration.

Catheter Obstruction

Catheter-related mechanical complications, including catheter obstruction are most commonly seen in the first 3 months after catheter implantation and are a leading cause of catheter failure (12). Normal position of the intra-abdominal coiled portions is in the pelvis (Figure 10.1). Obstruction can result from intra- or extra-luminal interference with the catheter, as well as from kinks or migration of the catheter.

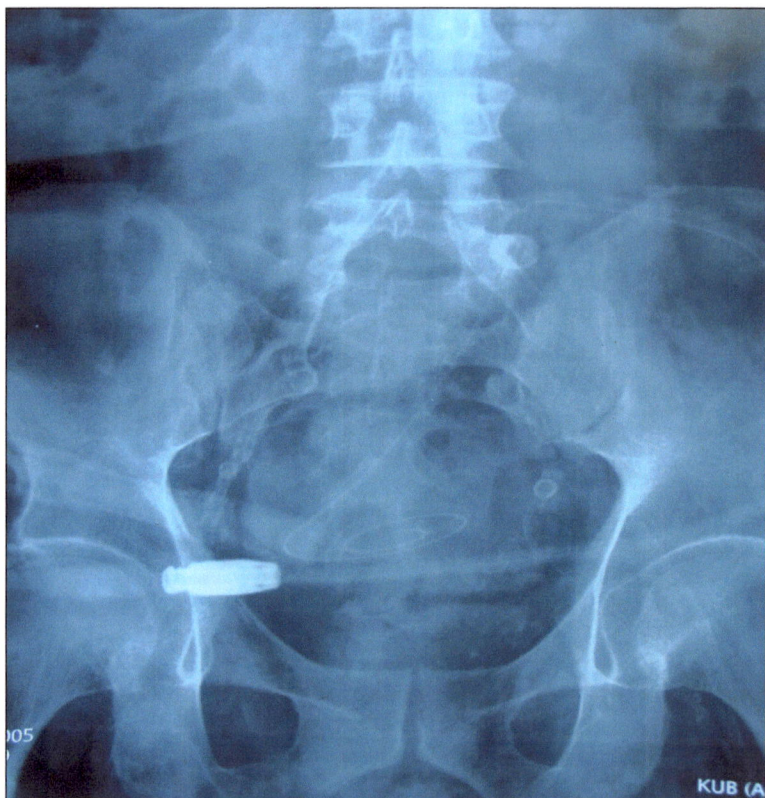

Figure 10.1. Abdominal X-ray Showing Normal Catheter Position
The coiled portion of the catheter rests in the pelvis.

Extra-luminal Obstruction

With an extra-luminal obstruction, dialysate inflow may remain intact. Constipation is a very common cause of external catheter obstruction. Patients in the immediate postoperative period are at high risk for developing constipation due to several contributing factors that act in concert. They include manipulation of the bowel during catheter implantation, poor oral intake, physical inactivity, and routine use of narcotics for pain control. Distended loops of bowel caused by constipation will wrap around the catheter, blocking the side holes in the intra-abdominal segment of the catheter or dislocating the tip of catheter out of the pelvic area and impairing catheter outflow (1). Thus, constipation should always be expected and a mild laxative should be given routinely starting the day before surgery and continuing for

2–3 days after the pain medication is stopped. Indeed, the ISPD recommends using a preoperative bowel regimen to prevent constipation (13). If obstruction persists after appropriate treatment for constipation, a plain radiograph of the abdomen should be obtained to confirm the catheter position, as migration is the second common cause of poor outflow (Figure 10.2). While inappropriate catheter placement can occasionally cause catheter outflow problems, migration of the PD catheter is more often the cause. Migration is often associated with poor orientation of the catheter's tunnel, resulting in misdirection of the catheter's intra-abdominal segment as it enters the abdomen. Migration of the catheter tip is more common when the catheter incision site is placed on the right side, because of the upward peristaltic movement of the ascending colon. Conversely, catheters that have migrated to the left upper quadrant (Figure 10.3) may spontaneously reposition themselves, influenced by the favorable downward peristalsis on the left side. During the initial catheter placement, correct alignment of the catheter in the rectus as it exits the abdomen reduces the risk of later dislodgment. The proper intra-abdominal alignment of the catheter is detailed in Chapter 2 (Figures 2.28, 2.29, 2.31, 2.40).

Fluoroscopic repositioning with a stiff guidewire has limited success; achieving restored acceptable flow and catheter position in only 30–50% of the cases. Recurrence of migration is common and usually requires reinsertion with special attention to tunnel orientation. Laparoscopic surgery to reposition and secure the intra-abdominal tip of the catheter in the true pelvis with a stitch can prevent or correct this complication (14,15) (Figure 4.15). Use of a specially designed catheter with a titanium weight at the distal end has been shown to prevent catheter migration (Figure 5.13).

External catheter obstruction can also be caused by adhesions from prior peritonitis or surgery, which may trap the catheter in a loculated compartment. Laparoscopic or surgical lysis of adhesions, or catheter repositioning or replacement may be necessary. (Figures 4.14–4.17)

Omental wrapping is another cause of extra-luminal obstruction of PD catheters. Attempts at fluoroscopic repositioning with a guidewire usually have limited success. Permanent corrective intervention requires a minilaparotomy (infra-umbilical midline incision) or laparoscopy to remove the omental tissue off the catheter and possibly suture placement to redirect the catheter into the pelvis (16–18). These surgical techniques are discussed in Chapter 4 (Figures 4.16, 4.17).

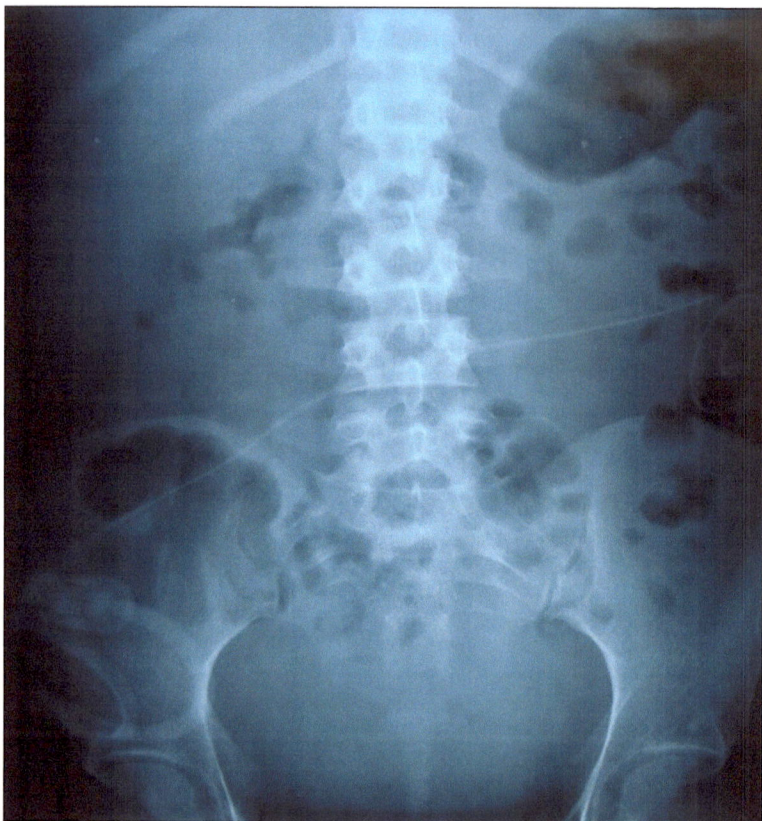

Figure 10.2. Abdominal X-ray Showing a Migrated Catheter
The tip of the catheter has migrated out of the pelvis to the left side of the abdomen; an improper tunnel and constipation are the causes identified.

Intra-luminal Obstruction

The lumen of the PD catheter can be blocked internally by fibrin or blood clot. Intra-luminal obstruction usually presents as failure of the PD catheter during infusion. Although usually ineffective, thrombolytic therapy may dissolve the clot if treatment with saline irrigation is ineffective. In persistent cases, direct intervention using a rigid guidewire or brush under fluoroscopic control may be attempted. In most situations, surgical or laparoscopic intervention becomes the treatment of choice.

Total obstruction—associated with no inflow (despite some force) and no drainage—is likely the result of a kink in the catheter. Upon confirmation, the problem can be solved with manipulation using a flexible probe, or if persistent, by laparoscopic or surgical repositioning.

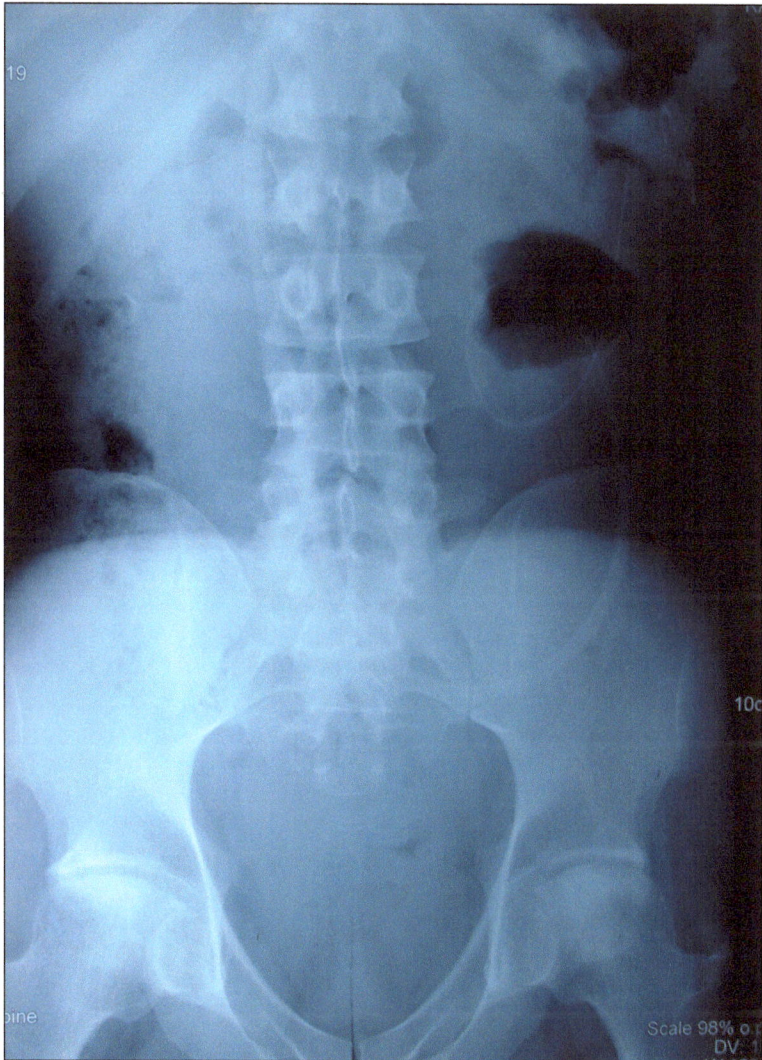

Figure 10.3. Abdominal X-ray Showing a Dislodged Catheter
The tip of the catheter has migrated out of the pelvis to the left upper quadrant of the abdomen.

Hydrothorax

Hydrothorax is a well-described but uncommon complication of PD, reported in 1–10% of cases (19–21). It typically occurs early in the course of therapy and is usually attributable to congenital defects or localized absence of muscle fibers of the diaphragm (22–25). As a result, the increase in IAP from instillation of PD fluid can prompt trickling of fluid from the peritoneal cavity into the pleural space, causing hydrothorax (26). (Figure 10.4)

Hydrothorax is more commonly seen in women; the reasons are unclear. Stretching of the diaphragm during pregnancy has been suggested as one plausible mechanism (23). Similarly, patients with polycystic kidney disease are more prone to develop hydrothorax (27). Hydrothorax usually develops on the right side, possibly because the heart and pericardium in the left hemithorax prevent flux of fluid across the left hemidiaphragm (23). Hydrothorax has rarely been observed on the left side, or both sides (28). In extremely rare occasions, pericardial effusion can ensue from communication of fluids between peritoneum and pericardial cavities (29,30).

Usually hydrothorax develops early in the course of PD if there are preexisting defects allowing communication of fluids between the peritoneal cavity and right pleural space. Conversely, hydrothorax may develop months to years after PD initiation, when minute diaphragmatic defects cause a 1-way passage of small volumes of fluid from the peritoneal to the pleural cavity, resulting in a slow buildup of hydrothorax over time. Though rare, an episode of peritonitis can damage the fragile barrier between the 2 cavities, triggering development of hydrothorax (31) (Figure 10.4).

This patient initiated PD about a week prior to presenting with shortness of breath. Examination of pleural fluid showed the fluid to be transudate with very high glucose content. Further evaluation revealed several defects in the diaphragm, which lead to pleura peritoneal communication.

About 25% of patients, particularly those with small defects, are asymptomatic and hydrothorax is diagnosed during a routine physical examination including chest x-rays. Most patients usually present with dyspnea and inadequate UF. Unlike patients with fluid overload, dyspnea worsens with use of higher strength dextrose solutions because of the increase in IAP (from increased UF with high dextrose solutions), causing increased efflux of fluid into pleural space. Therefore, in cases with worsening dyspnea while using hypertonic dialysate, and a decrease in effluent volume, hydrothorax should be considered.

Diagnosis of PD-associated hydrothorax is suggested by the presence of a pleural effusion particularly on the right side. A pleural fluid glucose concentration of >500 mg/dl or at least 50 mg/dl higher than a concurrent plasma sample is highly suggestive of a pleuroperitoneal communication. Additionally a low protein concentration of the pleural fluid is consistent with PD-induced hydrothorax. Pleuroperitoneal communication is best localized with an injection of methylene blue dye or radioisotopes into the peritoneal cavity followed by thoracentesis (blue staining of pleural fluid) or scintigram, respectively. However, intraperitoneal methylene blue can lead to chemical peritonitis or the blue staining may be too faint, causing false negative results. Isotopic scanning involves instillation of 3 mCi of technetium-labeled albumin or 10 mCi of sulfur colloid into the peritoneal cavity followed by a scan of pleural cavity (32,33). False negative results can occur with isotopic scanning in some instances. Other methods to detect peritoneal defects include non-contrast peritoneography, magnetic resonance imaging, and direct visualization using video thoracoscopy. Experience with these techniques is limited. (34)

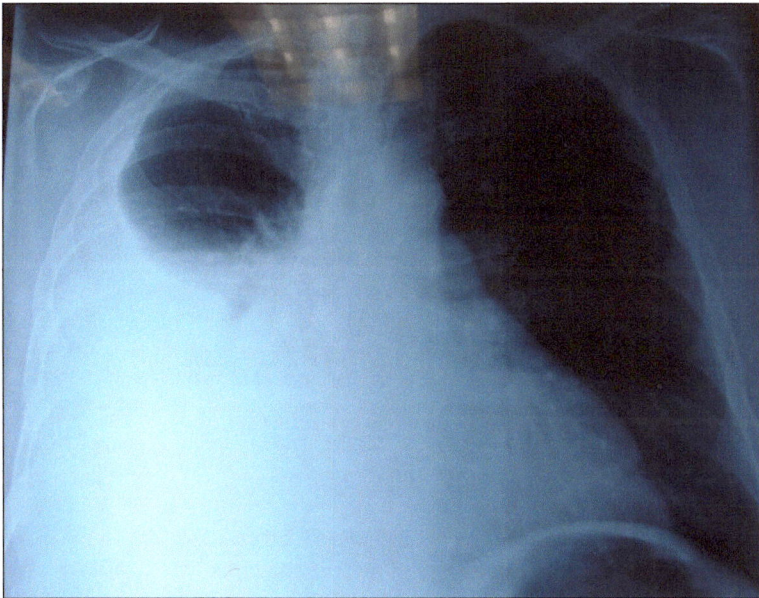

Figure 10.4. Chest x-ray of Patient who presented with Shortness of Breath

The presence of a hydrothorax precludes PD unless the pleuroperitoneal communication is obliterated. In recent years, significant progress has been made in the treatment of peritoneal leaks into pleural space allowing restoration of successful PD therapy.

In patients who present with severe respiratory distress, therapeutic thoracentesis offers immediate relief. Typically, 2–4 liters of fluid is drained. In most cases, discontinuation of PD leads to resolution of the pleural effusion in 2–4 weeks (21). In patients, with adequate RRF, who want to continue on PD, several treatment options are available. PD can be resumed using a nighttime cycler, with low volumes, in a supine position, for 4–6 weeks; similar to the description above for the treatment of dialysate leaks. (35). Another sometimes successful option includes disruption of PD for 4–6 weeks to allow pleural defects to heal before resuming low-volume PD exchanges in a supine position (36).

When conservative measures fail, surgical and interventional options include pleurodesis with infusion of irritants, such as oxytetracycline, talc, autologous blood, and other irritants (such as OK-432, a preparation from hemolytic streptococci; and Nocardia rubra cell wall skeleton). Fibrin glue injected into the pleural space has been used (37). Surgical, video-assisted thoracoscopic (VATS) closure of the diaphragmatic defect is the definitive, and usually successful, procedure (37).

Pain

Pain is common following surgical implantation of the catheter. Mild superficial pain at the incision site as well as deep pain associated with traction of the bowel and omentum is frequently experienced by patients in the immediate postoperative period. Later on, patients may experience pain during dialysate infusion or drainage. Moderate to severe pain experienced immediately after infusion suggests irritation of the peritoneum by the low pH of conventional dialysis solutions. It is self-limited and resolves in 2–4 weeks. Occasionally, addition of lidocaine (50 mg/ 2L of dialysate) or bicarbonate (10–20 ml of 50% bicarbonate) may help to relieve the pain (38). Using the novel high-pH solutions (bicarbonate based or amino-acid based dialysate solutions with higher pH) has been reported to resolve infusion pain resulting from the usage of low pH dialysate solutions. These high-pH solutions are not approved by the FDA for use in the USA but are commonly used in Europe and elsewhere. Localized pain during infusion may also ensue from irritation caused by the catheter tip rubbing against the pelvic wall or intra-abdominal organs like the bladder or rectum. Adhesions around the catheter restricting flow into a small compartment or suction created by the jet of rapid flow of solution can also result in infusion pain. The pain often resolves by moving the tip of the catheter to another location or replacing the catheter with a shorter one. If the pain persists, abdominal imaging is required to assess the location of the catheter. Laparoscopic or open surgical lysis of the adhesions or replacement of the catheter may be required to relieve intractable infusion pain.

Pain during drainage of the effluent is usually experienced in patients who start PD exchanges with a cycler. Pain can be caused by the suction created by the cycler during the dialysate outflow. Constipation or other causes of outflow obstruction described above can aggravate the pain. When outflow pain is experienced, constipation should always be ruled out first. If constipation is present, an appropriate bowel regimen should be instituted. In the absence of constipation, other causes of outflow obstruction should be pursued and treated as described above. If there is no evidence of outflow obstruction, a 90–95% tidal PD should be instituted. This entails removing only 90–95% of the infused dialysate during the initial exchanges and removing the remainder of the dialysate with the last exchange. This will create less negative suction force with the initial PD exchanges and would relieve the pain during PD drainage.

Bleeding and Hemoperitoneum

Bleeding and hemoperitoneum can result during surgery or in the immediate postoperative period. It usually results from laceration of the abdominal wall or intra-abdominal blood vessels. Postoperative bleeding will require immediate intervention and ligation of the bleeding vessel through either laparoscopy or laparotomy. Venous bleeding may be more difficult to identify and control since veins do not have a muscularis layer. The recommended approach depends on the severity of the bleeding.

Later in the course of PD, bleeding manifests as hemoperitoneum. Even a small amount of blood (2–4 ml) can render the dialysate blood tinged enough to cause concern to the patient and the physician. The most common cause of hemoperitoneum is menstruation, accounting for more than 1/3 of the episodes (39–41). Ruptured ovarian cysts and mid-cycle bleeding during ovulation are other common causes of hemoperitoneum in women (39–41). Most of these cases are benign, but sometimes bleeding may be severe enough to require a blood transfusion or hormone therapy to stop the bleeding.

In non-menstruating women and in men, hemoperitoneum is not that common and warrants careful workup including imaging procedures and surgical consultation if indicated. A myriad of causes can result in hemoperitoneum in this patient population. They include peritonitis, cholecystitis, pancreatitis, injury or rupture of abdominal organs, malfunction of abdominal instrumentation, faulty procedures, and malignant tumors. Occasionally, hemoperitoneum can develop from pressure necrosis of vascular structures around the catheter. Recurrent hemoperitoneum may be associated with encapsulating peritoneal sclerosis (39). Rupture of cysts in patients with polycystic kidney disease or patients with acquired renal cysts can be associated with hemoperitoneum.

The management of hemoperitoneum includes anticoagulation with heparin (500 units/L) to prevent blood clotting in the catheter lumen. Intraperitoneal heparin, in this dose, does not cause bleeding or systemic anticoagulation, and should be used as long as the dialysate has visible blood or fibrin. Rapid exchanges of PD fluid at the time of initial presentation can facilitate washing out the collected blood in the peritoneum and may help to prevent catheter blockage. Surgical or laparoscopic intervention may be needed in intractable cases.

Infectious Complications

Infections involving PD catheters can be classified into three categories, depending on the segment of the catheter involved: exit site infections, tunnel infections and peritonitis. The treatment varies with the location of infection and the etiology.

Exit-site Infections

Exit-site infections present with erythema and purulent drainage from the skin exit site. Skin bacteria are the cause. Untreated, these infections progress to tunnel infections and even peritonitis. Simple infections without drainage are treated with antibiotics and improved local hygiene (42,43). Exit-site infections involving the subcutaneous cuff can be treated with simple drainage of the site and externalization of the subcutaneous cuff, which is then "shaved" to remove all cuff material as a source for harboring bacteria. This effectively converts a 2-cuff catheter into a 1-cuff catheter. Drainage and cuff externalization cannot be performed with single-cuff catheters.

Tunnel Infections

Tunnel infections typically present in conjunction with exit-site infections, but can occur alone, usually with abscess formation. Patients may have tenderness or erythema overlying the catheter tract. Tunnel infections are treated with antibiotics. If an abscess is present, an incision and drainage must be performed, and the subcutaneous Dacron cuff shaved. In 7–10 days, the catheter can be re-routed to a new exit site.

Peritonitis

Peritonitis represents the most common cause of PD failure and subsequent conversion to HD. Gram-positive organisms are the etiology of a majority of all episodes of peritonitis (44%), with coagulase negative staphylococcus being the most frequent gram-positive organism of all (44). Twenty-five percent of peritonitis episodes are due to gram-negative organisms and 20% of cases are culture negative. A center's peritonitis rate should not exceed 1 episode per 18 months as recommended by the ISPD (43). Higher rates should prompt a review of techniques and re-education of both patients and staff to ensure that technique is not contributing to the high rates of peritonitis. The routes of peritoneal infection include bacterial penetration through the catheter wall— externally or along the tunnel (35–50%), contamination at the exit site (15–25%), and from intra-abdominal sources (20%). Bacteria translocations through an intact bowel can occur in the presence of colonoscopy, colitis/diarrhea, or even constipation. Though rare, a perforated intestine (i.e. from a toothpick, appendicitis, colon cancer, inflammatory disease, or complication from laparoscopy) can also cause peritonitis and should be suspected in the appropriate clinical setting.

The most common presentation of peritonitis in patients on PD is abdominal pain with a cloudy, sometimes bloody effluent. A clear effluent does not rule out peritonitis and a cloudy effluent alone does not always indicate the patient has peritonitis. Cloudy effluents are also associated with malignancies, chemical peritonitis, or a sample from a "dry" abdomen. If peritonitis is suspected, empiric antibiotics should be started after sending a sample of peritoneal fluid for evaluation. Antibiotic selection should cover both gram-positive and gram-negative organisms. Intraperitoneal administration is superior to intravenous dosing (43). In diagnosing peritonitis, an effluent with a white blood cell count of more than 100/mm3 with at least 50% polymorphonuclear cells is highly suggestive. Even if the cell count does not reach 100/mm3, as in the instance of a "dry" abdomen, a proportion greater than 50% polymorphonuclear cells suggests peritonitis. Once culture results are available, antibiotic therapy is directed to treat the identified organisms. Episodes of uncomplicated peritonitis are not an indication for catheter removal but refractory peritonitis (failure to improve after 5 days of appropriate antibiotics) and relapsing peritonitis (recurrence after 4 weeks of treatment) often require catheter removal. Coagulase-negative staphylococcal infections can lead to the formation of a biofilm that results in recurrent peritonitis—these catheters should also be removed. Fungal and polymicrobial peritonitis are indications for prompt catheter removal.

Unusual and often difficult cases require specific measures including special tools, operating room equipment, as well as surgical and radiologic skill. Examples of such cases are PD fluid leaking into the pleural space, unexplained chest pain, bleeding into the abdomen, perforated intestines, and pregnancies.

SUMMARY

Despite evidence of improved survival and quality of life compared to HD, PD is associated with significant morbidity over the lifetime of the catheter. Careful evaluation of each patient and a surgical plan are integral parts of the multidisciplinary teamwork involved in caring for patients with ESRD. Catheter function rates as high as 91% at 3 years can be accomplished with proper preoperative planning, safely performed surgery, and careful patient management (13).

REFERENCES

1. Davidson IJA. *Access for Dialysis: surgical and radiologic procedures.* 2nd ed. Austin, TX: Landes Bioscience. Third edition available for preview at www.ingemardavidson.com.

2. Saha TC, Singh H. Noninfectious complications of peritoneal dialysis. *South Med J* 2007; 100: 54.

3. Van Dijk CMA, Ledesma SG, Teitelbaum I. Patient characteristics associated with defects of the peritoneal cavity boundary. *Perit Dial Int* 2005; 25: 367-73.

4. Del Peso G, Bajo MA, Costero O, et al. Risk factors for abdominal wall complications in peritoneal dialysis patients. *Perit Dial Int* 2003; 23: 249–254.

5. Van Dijk CM, Ledesma SG, Teitelbaum I. Patient characteristics associated with defects of the peritoneal cavity boundary. *Perit Dial Int* 2005; 25: 367–373.

6. Tzamaloukas AH, Gibel LJ, Eisenberg B, et al. Early and late peritoneal dialysate leaks in patients on CAPD. *Adv Perit Dial* 1990; 6:64–70.

7. Twardowski ZJ, Tully RJ, Nichols WK. Computerized tomography CT in the diagnosis of subcutaneous leak sites during continuous ambulatory peritoneal dialysis. *Perit Dial Bull* 1984; 4:163–166.

8. Schultz SG, Harmon TM, Nachtnebel KL. Computerized tomographic scanning with intraperitoneal contrast enhancement in a CAPD patient with localized edema. *Perit Dial Bull* 1984; 4:253–254.

9. Twardowski ZJ, Tully RJ, Ersoy FF & Dedhia NM. Computerized tomography with and without intraperitoneal contrast for determination of intra-abdominal fluid distribution and diagnosis of complications in peritoneal dialysis patients. *ASAIO Trans* 1990; 36:95–103.

10. Kopecky RT, Foymeyer PA, Witanowski LS, Thomas FD. Complications of continuous ambulatory peritoneal dialysis: diagnostic value of peritoneal scintigraphy. *Am J Kidney Dis* 1987; 136:123–132.

11. Joffe P. Peritoneal dialysis catheter leakage treated with fibrin glue. *Nephrol Dial Transplant* 1993; 8: 474-6.

12. Singh N, Davidson I, Minhajuddin A, et al: Risk factors associated with peritoneal dialysis catheter survival: a 9-year single-center study in 315 patients. *J Vasc Access* 2010; 11: 316.

13. Gokal R, Alexander S, Ash S, et al. Peritoneal catheters and exit-site practices toward optimum peritoneal access: 1998 update. *Perit Dial Int* 1998; 18: 11-33.

14. Ogunc G. Malfunctioning peritoneal dialysis catheter and accompanying surgical pathology repaired by laparoscopic surgery. *Perit Dial Int* 2002; 22: 454-62.

15. Dantoine T, Benevent D, Boudet R, Lagarde C, Charmes JP, Leroux-Robert C. Front-loading a peritoneal dialysis catheter prevents its migration in elderly patients. *Perit Dial Int* 2002; 22: 528-31.

16. Santarelli S, Zeiler M, Marinelli R, et al. Videolaparoscopy as rescue therapy and placement of peritoneal dialysis catheters: a thirty-two case single centre experience. *Nephrol Dial Transplant* 2006; 21: 1348.

17. Crabtree JH, Fishman A. Selective performance of prophylactic omentopexy during laparoscopic implantation of peritoneal dialysis catheters. *Surg Laparoscop Endoscop Percutan Tech* 2003; 13: 180.

18. Zadrozny D, Draczkowski T, Lichodziejewska-Niemierko K. Two-millimeter minisite mini-laparoscopy for rescue of dysfunctional continuous ambulatory peritoneal dialysis catheters. *Surg Laparosc Endosc Percutan Tech* 1999; 9: 369.

19. Duffy JP, Allen SM, Matthews HR. Hydrothorax due to dialysate leakage. *Clin Nephrol* 1994; 42: 65.

20. Garcia Ramon R, Carrasco AM. Hydrothorax in peritoneal dialysis. *Perit Dial Int* 1998; 18: 5–10.

21. Nomoto Y, Suga T, Nakajima K, et al. Acute hydrothorax in continuous ambulatory peritoneal dialysis – a collaborative study of 161 centers. *Am J Nephrol* 1989; 9: 363–367.

22. Chow CC, Sung JY, Cheung CK, Hamilton-Wood C, Lai KN. Massive hydrothorax in continuous ambulatory peritoneal dialysis: diagnosis, management and review of the literature. *N Z Med J* 1988; 101: 475–477.

23. Lieberman F, Hidemura R, Peters R, Reynolds T. Pathogenesis and treatment of hydrothorax complicating cirrhosis with ascites. *Ann Intern Med* 1966; 64: 341–351.

24. Boeschoten EW, Krediet RT, Roos CM, Kloek JJ, Schipper ME, Arisz L. Leakage of dialysate across the diaphragm: an important complication of continuous ambulatory peritoneal dialysis. *Neth J Med* 1986; 29: 242–246.

25. Gagnon RF, Daniels E. The persisting pneumatoenteric recess and the infracardiac bursa: possible role in the pathogenesis of right hydrothorax complicating peritoneal dialysis. *Adv Perit Dial* 2004; 20: 132–136.

26. Szeto CC, Chow KM. Pathogenesis and management of hydrothorax complicating peritoneal dialysis. *Curr Opin Pulm Med* 2004; 10: 315–319.

27. Fletcher S, Turney JH, Brownjohn AM. Increased incidence of hydrothorax complicating peritoneal dialysis in patients with adult polycystic kidney disease. *Nephrol Dial Transplant* 1994; 9: 832–833.

28. Sun SS, Kao CH. Unusual bilateral peritoneopleural communication associated with cirrhotic ascites: detected by TC-99m sulphur colloid peritoneoscintigraphy. *Kaohsiung J Med Sci* 2000; 16: 539–541.

29. Hou CH, Tsai TJ, Hsu KL. Peritoneopericardial communication after pericardiocentesis in a patient on continuous ambulatory peritoneal dialysis with dialysis pericarditis. *Nephron* 1994; 68: 125–127.

30. Nather S, Anger H, Koall W, et al. Peritoneal leak and chronic pericardial effusion in a CAPD patient. *Nephrol Dial Transplant* 1996; 11: 1155–1158.

31. Gagnon RF, Thirlweil M, Arzoumanian A, Mehio A. Systemic amyloidosis involving the diaphragm and acute massive hydrothorax during peritoneal dialysis. *Clin Nephrol* 2002; 57: 474–479.

32. Cory DA, Stephens BA, Herman PR. Massive hydrothorax complicating continuous ambulatory peritoneal dialysis. *Clin Nucl Med* 1993; 18: 526.

33. Contreras-Puertas P, Benitez-Sanchez M, Jimenez-Heffernan A, Rebollo-Aguirre A, Cruz-Munoz S. Hydrothorax in continuous ambulatory peritoneal dialysis: peritoneoscintigraphy in a case of spontaneous closure of pleuroperitoneal communication. *Clin Nucl Med* 2002; 27: 208–209.

34. Prischl FC, Muhr T, Seiringer EM, et al. Magnetic resonance imaging of the peritoneal cavity among peritoneal dialysis patients, using the dialysate as 'contrast medium'. *J Am Soc Nephrol* 2002; 13: 197–203.

35. Christidou F, Vayonas G. Recurrent acute hydrothorax in a CAPD patient: successful management with small volumes of dialysate. *Perit Dial Int* 1995; 15: 389.

36. Ing A, Rutland J, Kalowski S. Spontaneous resolution of hydrothorax in continuous ambulatory peritoneal dialysis. *Nephron* 1992; 61: 247–248.

37. Tang S, Chui WH, Tang AW, et al. Video-assisted thoracoscopic talc pleurodesis is effective for maintenance of peritoneal dialysis in acute hydrothorax complicating peritoneal dialysis. *Nephrol Dial Transplant* 2003; 18: 804-8.

38. Ahrens TS, Prentice D, Kleinpell R. Critical Care Nursing Certification. Fifth edition, *The McGraw-Hill* 2008; PP 569-583.

39. Greenberg A, Bernardini J, Piraino BM, Johnston JR, Perlmutter JA. Hemoperitoneum complicating chronic peritoneal dialysis: single-center experience and literature review. *Am J Kidney Dis* 1992; 19: 252–256.

40. Tse KC, Yip PS, Lam MF, et al. Recurrent hemoperitoneum complicating continuous ambulatory peritoneal dialysis. *Perit Dial Int* 2002; 22: 488–491.

41. Harnett JD, Gill D, Corbett L, Parfrey PS, Gault H. Recurrent hemoperitoneum in women receiving continuous ambulatory peritoneal dialysis. *Ann Intern Med* 1987; 107: 341–343.

42. Lew SQ, K Kaveh. Dialysis access related infections. *ASAIO J* 2000; 46: S6.

43. Li PKT, CC Szeto, B Piraino, et al. Peritoneal dialysis-related infections recommendations: 2010 update. *Perit Dial Int* 2010; 30: 393.

44. Kern EO, Newman LN, Cacho CP, et al. Abdominal catastrophe revisited: the risk and outcomes of enteric peritoneal contamination. *Perit Dial Int* 2002; 22: 323.

APPENDIX OF PERITONEAL DIALYSIS PRODUCTS CITED IN THIS VOLUME

Providing a complete list of commercially available PD products is difficult, considering that this book will be distributed worldwide. Here we cite only some of the main companies, which are holding copyrights or selling specific products that are cited in this Volume.

CATHETER	COMPANY
Tenckhoff catheter	Quinton, Seattle, WA, USA
Swan Neck catheter	Covidien, New Haven, CT, USA
Missouri Swan Neck catheter	Covidien, New Haven, CT, USA
Toronto Western Hospital catheter	Covidien, New Haven, CT, USA
Self-locating (Di Paolo) catheter	B. Braun Avitum, Melsungen, Germany
Pail-handle (Cruz) catheter	Corpak Med-Systems, Wheeling, IL, USA
Flex-Neck catheter	Janin Group - Medigroup, Oswego, IL, USA
Ash Advantage catheter	Janin Group - Medigroup, Oswego, IL, USA

TRANSFER SET	COMPANY
MiniCap Extended Life PD Transfer Set with Twist Cap	Baxter, Deerfield, IL, USA
PD Transfer Set Change Kit	Baxter, Deerfield, IL, USA
Dianeal Solution, Ultrabag System	Baxter, Deerfield, IL, USA
Stay-Safe System	Fresenius Medical Care, Waltham, MA, USA

CATHETER-COMPATIBLE SUPPLIES	COMPANY
Alcavis 50	Alcavis HDC, Gaithersburg, MD, USA
ExSept Plus	Alcavis HDC, Gaithersburg, MD, USA

CONTRIBUTORS AND THEIR AFFILIATIONS

Janet Bardsley, RN, CCRC
Home Modalities Nurse Coordinator
Barnes Jewish Dialysis Center
Washington University School of Medicine
4205 Forest Park Ave.
St. Louis, MO 63108
(314) 286-0804
jbardsle@dom.wustl.edu

Joanne M Bargman, MD, FRCPC
Professor of Medicine, University of Toronto
Staff Nephrologist, University Health Network
Director, Home Peritoneal Dialysis Unit
Director, Clinical Fellowship Program in Nephrology
at the University of Toronto
Toronto General Hospital
200 Elizabeth Street, 8N-840
Toronto, Ontario M5G 2C4 CANADA
+1 416 340-4804 (phone)
+1 416 340-4999 (fax)

Mary L Brandt, MD
Professor and Vice Chair, Michael E. DeBakey Department of Surgery
Baylor College of Medicine
Houston, TX 77030
brandt@bcm.edu
832-822-3135

Ingemar Davidson, MD, PhD
Professor of Surgery, Division of Transplant
UT Southwestern Medical Center
Parkland Memorial Hospital
5939 Harry Hines Blvd.
Dallas, TX 75390-8567
ingemardavidson@UTSouthwestern.edu
drd@ingemardavidson.com
214-645-7670

Maurizio Gallieni, MD
Director, Nephrology and Dialysis Unit
Ospedale San Carlo Borromeo, Milan - Italy
Coordinating Editor, Journal of Vascular Access
maurizio.gallieni@ sancarlo.mi.it
www.vascular-access.info
+390240222343

Kendle Frazier, CST
Operating Room
Forest Park Medical Center
11990 North Central Expressway
Dallas, TX 75243
972-234-1900

Christine Hwang, MD
Assistant professor of Surgery, Division of Transplant
UT Southwestern Medical Center
Parkland Memorial Hospital
5939 Harry Hines Blvd.
Dallas, TX 75390-8567
christine.hwang@UTSouthwestern.edu
214-645-7670

Shawna McMichael, RN
Home Modalities Nurse Coordinator
Barnes Jewish Dialysis Center
Washington University School of Medicine
4205 Forest Park Ave.
St. Louis, MO 63108
(314) 286-0847
smcmicha@dom.wustl.edu

Anil Paramesh, MD
Assistant Professor, Department of Surgery
Tulane University
1430 Tulane Avenue
New Orleans, LA 70112-2699
aparames@tulane.edu
504-988-2317

Eric Peden, MD
Methodist Hospital
DeBakey Heart & Vascular Center
6550 Fannin Street
Houston, TX 77030
EKPeden@tmhs.org
713-441-5200

Ramesh Saxena, MD, PhD
Professor of Medicine, Division of Nephrology
UT Southwestern Medical Center
Parkland Memorial Hospital
5939 Harry Hines Blvd.
Dallas TX 75390-8856
ramesh.saxena@UTSouthwestern.edu
214-648-2681

Daniel Scott, MD
Professor of Surgery, UT Southwestern Medical Center
Parkland Memorial Hospital
5939 Harry Hines Blvd.
Dallas, TX 75390-9031
daniel.scott@UTSouthwestern.edu
214-648-2677

Douglas Slakey, MD, MPH
Professor and Chair, Department of Surgery
Tulane University
1430 Tulane Avenue
New Orleans, LA 70112-2699
dslakey@tulane.edu
504-988-2317

Min C Yoo, MD
UT Southwestern Medical Center
Parkland Memorial Hospital
5939 Harry Hines Blvd.
Dallas, TX 75390-8567
mcyoo@utexas.edu
214-645-7670

DAVIDSON MEDICAL SERIES

VOLUME I

PERITONEAL DIALYSIS

Surgical Technique and Medical Management

EDITORS

INGEMAR DAVIDSON
MAURIZIO GALLIENI
RAMESH SAXENA

DAVIDSON MEDICAL SERIES

VOLUME II

HEMODIALYSIS

Surgical Technique and Medical Management

EDITORS

INGEMAR DAVIDSON
CHARMAINE LOK
JOHN ROSS

IN COLLABORATION WITH
JOHN R. ROSS, MD

DAVIDSON MEDICAL SERIES

VOLUME III

CENTRAL VENOUS ACCESS

Catheter Insertion Techniques in Dialysis and Oncology

EDITORS

INGEMAR DAVIDSON
MAURIZIO GALLIENI
ANTONIO LAGRECA
MAURO PITTIRUTI

DAVIDSON MEDICAL SERIES

VOLUME IV

VASCULAR ACCESS CASE REPORTS

Illustrated Surgical and Radiologic Interventional Techniques

EDITORS

INGEMAR DAVIDSON
BART DOLMATCH
JOHN ROSS

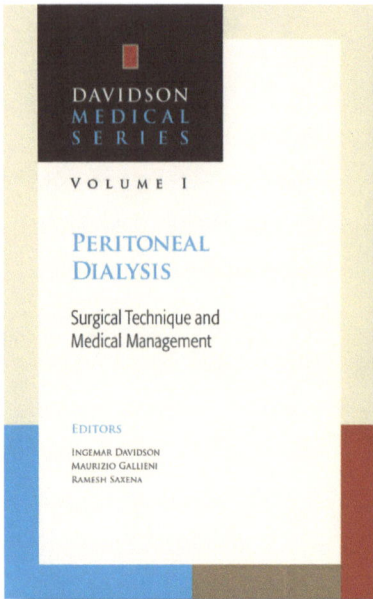

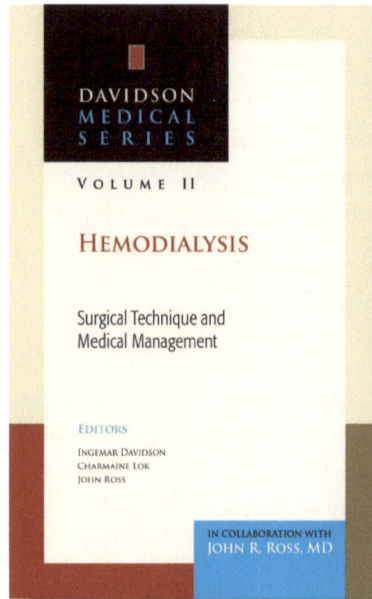

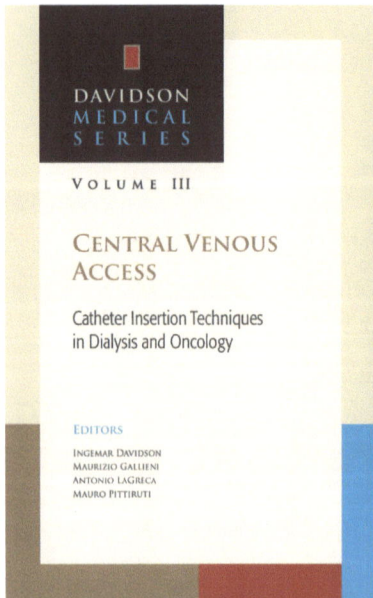

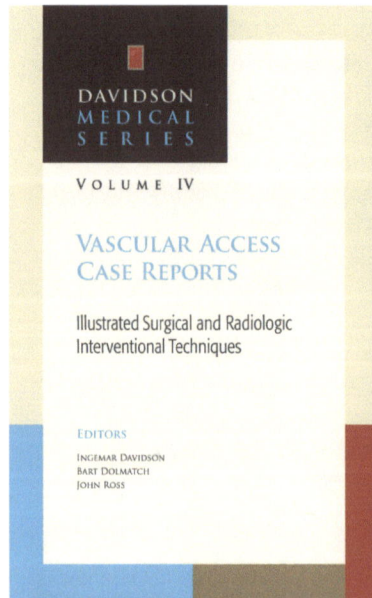

DAVIDSON MEDICAL SERIES BY DIVADI, LLC
WWW.INGEMARDAVIDSON.COM